MEDITATIONS
on Diabetes

STRENGTHENING
YOUR SPIRIT IN
EVERY SEASON

CATHERINE FESTE

American Diabetes Association.

Editor   Sherrye L. Landrum
Production Coordinator   Peggy M. Rote
Composition   Harlowe Typography, Inc.
Text and Cover Design   Wickham & Associates, Inc.

Printed in Canada
1 3 5 7 9 10 8 6 4 2

ADA titles may be purchased for business or promotional use or for special sales. For information, please write to: Lee M. Romano, Special Sales & Promotions, American Diabetes Association, 1660 Duke Street, Alexandria, Virginia 22314.

Library of Congress Cataloging-in-Publication Data

Feste, Catherine.
    Meditations on diabetes: strengthening your spirit in all seasons
/ Catherine Feste, with a foreword by Rachel Naomi Remen.
    p. cm.
    ISBN 1-58040-001-9
    1. Diabetes–Popular works.   2. Diabetes–Psychological aspects.
3. Diabetes–Quotations,maxins, etc.   I. Title.
RC660.4.F47   1999
616.4'62–dc21   98-45648
                                                 CIP

Dedication

I gratefully acknowledge my husband, Dale, and our son, John. Their love, support, and inspiration have helped me to cope with many challenges. Their presence in my life has been the Joy that has inspired me to manage diabetes. It is to these two gentle men of my heart that this book is lovingly dedicated.

Contents

Foreword

I
t is only quite recently that illness has been defined as a function of the body. At the beginnings of medicine, the shamans or medicine men defined illness not in terms of pathology but in terms of the soul. In this older wisdom, illness is "soul loss," a loss of direction, purpose, meaning, mystery, and awe. According to these ancients, the healing from illness required an attention to the realm of spirit, a recovery of the soul.

What then is spirit? Spirit is the basis for the value of every human life, the source of our dignity, and the foundation of our experience of integrity, despite bodily changes. The capacity for spiritual experience is so universal that every language has its own name for it: the Atman, the Neshuma, the Ra, the Ru-ach, the Divine Spark. We call this capacity the soul.

Illness and suffering draw the soul and its issues closer. Everything I have learned about spirit I have learned from listening to people with cancer in my work as a physician and from my long and personal experience with Crohn's disease, a chronic illness of the intestine.

These experiences have taught me that spirit is not just a human capacity, it is a human need. This seems especially true in times of loss, in times of illness and crisis. At such times, spirit is strength.

The pursuit of meaning is often the doorway to the spirit. The language of the soul is meaning. In the setting of a chronic illness, people instinctively reach for personal meaning, people who have never considered this dimension of life before. Meaning helps us to see in the dark. It strengthens the will to live in us.

Our sense of the meaning of a common event is as unique as our fingerprints: an illness like diabetes will mean something different to every person who is touched by it. Many years ago when I went to medical school, the meaning of an illness was seen as irrelevant. But we did not know much about healing then. Our focus was on cure. While cure happens to the body, healing happens to the whole person. Many things that are beyond cure can still heal. I suppose one might even say that there is a healthy way to have a disease, a way to use this difficult experience to come to know intimately the value and meaning of your life.

Experiencing spirit and meaning does not require us to live differently. Many of us already live far more meaningful lives than we realize. Experiencing meaning often requires a shift in perspective, the development of new eyes. Finding meaning is about seeing beyond the superficial and the obvious to the essential. Seeing the ordinary and the familiar in new ways. Meaning does not change the events of our lives, it changes our experience of those events. It may be the difference between seeing yourself as a victim and seeing yourself as a hero.

Through illness, people may come to know themselves for the first time, to recognize not only who they really are but what really matters. Illness shuffles the hierarchy of our values like a deck of cards. Often a value that has been on the bottom of the deck for years turns out to be the top card. In illness, people abandon values they inherited with their family name, values that they have never questioned before, and uncover ways of living far more genuine and unique. Often these ways are also more soul-infused. In all the years that I have listened to people with cancer, no one has ever said to me that if they died, they would miss their Mercedes, even though such a car and all that it represents has been the focus of their lives for many years. This shift may represent a kind of healing.

Illness often naturally initiates a movement toward greater wholeness. In the 25 years that I have been a physician to people with cancer, I have witnessed this many times over. I have been with people as they have discovered in themselves an unexpected strength, a courage beyond what they would have thought possible, an unsuspected sense of compassion, and a capacity for love far deeper than they had ever dreamed.

When I first became ill with my own chronic illness more than 45 years ago, I felt profoundly diminished, different, and even ashamed. I had not known then that what challenges the body can evolve and strengthen the soul. I had focused on the curing of my body. It took years for me to recognize the movement toward wholeness that had happened in me while my attention was elsewhere—to know that it is possible to live a good life even if it is not an easy life.

Curing is about the recovery of the body. Healing is about the recovery of the soul. Science cures us. Meaning heals us. Some years ago I wrote this poem about my own experience of illness:

O
Body!
For 45 years,
1,573 experts with a combined
14,355 years of training

have failed
to
cure
your
wounds.

Deep inside,
I
am
whole.

The capacity for spirit and meaning are a part of our birthright as human beings. My experience as both physician and patient has led me to believe that illness is often an awakening and a spiritual path. There are many ways to travel this path, to move toward our wholeness, and strengthen the innate spirit in us. *Meditations on Diabetes* offers us a wide variety of such approaches, and I am honored to be asked to introduce this book to you. It is a book of wisdom for the path, and a gift to those whose lives have been touched by diabetes. It will help anyone who reads it to use the experience of illness to deepen and enrich the experience of life.

Rachel Naomi Remen, MD

Author, *Kitchen Table Wisdom: Stories that Heal*

Acknowledgments

From the beginning, this project has been surrounded by love and guided by a wide and wonderful variety of angels. Their contributions included serving as a sounding board as I tried out the thoughts that became foundational to the book. Some of them served as reviewers and shared helpful comments and insights. Several of the messages I used came from messenger angels listed here. I acknowledge these people and their contributions to this book and to my life: Mark Anderson, Anne Carlson, Mary Casey, Sheila Folkestad, Lyle Gerard, Dick and Diana Guthrie, Mary Jackson, Delores Kanten, Judy Louden, Terry Morehouse, Jan Norman, Jan Olson, Ginny Peragallo-Dittko, Kathy Plumb, Ellen Reeder, Dawn Satterfield, Rich and Linda Sedgwick, Dan Schindler, Jen Smith, Ruth Stricker, and Nancy Youngdahl.

Special thanks to Sherrye Landrum, my wonderful editor, whose enthusiasm, encouragement, and guidance were critical to the writing of this

book. And, a special word of thanks to my long-
time friend and mentor, Bob Esbjornson. He
shared his important perspectives as religion professor, medical ethicist, husband, and father of
people who have diabetes, and he shared his beautiful soul. Thanks, Esbj.

For their remarkable and inspiring leadership
in the field of healing and spirituality, I owe a
heartfelt and profound "thank you" to Dr. MaryJo
Kreitzer, Director of Complementary Care and The
Center for Spirituality and Healing at the Univer-
sity of Minnesota; Dr. Dean Ornish, author, *Love &
Survival* and *Dr. Dean Ornish's Program for Reversing
Heart Disease* and Clinical Professor of Medicine,
University of California, San Francisco School of
Medicine; and Dr. Rachel Naomi Remen, author,
Kitchen Table Wisdom: Stories That Heal, cofounder
and Medical Director, Commonweal Cancer Help
Program and Associate Clinical Professor of Family
and Community Medicine, University of California, San Francisco School of Medicine. They are my
heroes. They are the true pioneers whose courage
and conviction have opened new pathways to healing. All of us are the beneficiaries of their devotion,
dedication, wisdom, and hard work. Their Being has
been a blessing to both my life and my work. Their
spirits strengthened mine, and I am forever grateful.

Introduction

When I was a small child, one of the prayers that I said asked God's help so I could be "sweet and gentle in all the disappointments in life." Pretty quickly, I had my own definition of disappointments. My father died when I was nine years old, and I was diagnosed with diabetes when I was ten. I've been talking with God for a long time now through all sorts of disappointments. My definition of sweet and gentle has taken on overtones of tough and resilient, but my prayer is the same.

I learned about courage, faith, and determination from my mother. The day after Dad's funeral, she invited my 12-year-old brother and me to join her as she drove the car around the block. She had never driven a car before. Her message was clear: Life goes on. Each of us has things to learn and things to do while we are here that no one else can do for us.

Hungry to know more about my father, I seized every story and every piece of evidence that might tell me something about him. I was given a prayer book that he had received from the Methodist Church Sunday School. I read it slowly and repeatedly, wondering what disappointments it had helped him to bear. Had he taken it to Europe when he served in World War II? Had he pondered its principles while he built his law practice?

I learned more about his family and his grandmother when I was given her Bible. As I carefully leafed through the worn and tattered pages, I saw that she had read with frequency the books that I love—most notably, the Psalms. In the back of her Bible, I found a tithing covenant that she signed in 1929. A widow with four young sons, she committed to a ten-percent tithe to the church at the beginning of the Great Depression. These stories became woven into the fabric of my life as I sought the courage to live with the challenges that life was presenting to me.

Ten months after Dad died, I was diagnosed with diabetes. Back in the 1950s, people were hospitalized for a week or ten days with that diagnosis. I had a lot of time to think about what was going on—including the reason I was in the pediatrics (Peds) ward of a small Wisconsin hospital. I had just settled in at summer camp for a week. I was elated to have been assigned a top bunk, but I never got to sleep in it. During evening games, I fell and broke my arm. In the hospital, I had a routine blood test that showed a very high blood sugar. So, I had to hang out in the Peds ward for ten more days.

I assessed my roommates. The girl in the bed next to mine had "water on the brain." That was all I knew and that she had a very large head. A boy who had a ruptured appendix occupied the next bed. And in the isolation room lay a little boy who'd broken his leg. Now he was immobilized with a pin through his thigh and his leg in traction. By the time my arm was in a cast, my blood sugar was responding to insulin, and I felt fine. I decided I was much better off than the other kids, so I spent my days reading stories to them.

On the night of the fourth of July, a group of men dressed as clowns carrying helium-filled balloons came to visit the Peds ward. They came down to my bed first because I was at the end of the row. As a clown extended a balloon to me, I refused it saying, "You don't have to give me a balloon. I just have a broken arm and diabetes. I'm not sick."

My mother helped me form that attitude from the beginning. A few days earlier, when I had asked her what it meant to have diabetes, she'd said, "Diabetes means that we're going to learn so much about good nutrition. We're going to live such a healthy lifestyle that the whole family will benefit. And you will always be a stronger, more self-disciplined person." Not until I became engaged to be married did Mother reveal that when she had practiced injections on an orange, tears had streamed down her face. Her positive attitude had masked a great deal of pain.

These early experiences shaped me in ways that are still revealing themselves. I know this because I have continued to observe my life and look for the different threads that appear and reappear in it. Perhaps I must thank my early disappointments for encouraging the deep thinking in which I engaged at a young age. I suspect that all children do think about the meaning of life, but I am grateful that this trait became part of my adult lifestyle, a meditative lifestyle. I became—and remain—a seeker of meaning.

I have made some discoveries over the years. I believe that if life has a meaning we can live with comfortably, then we are less stressed. I believe that the philosophy we live by shapes our attitudes and directs our behavior. We arrive at meanings and philosophies through thinking. In particular,

I believe that thinking about stories (our own and others') helps us find meaning and define our philosophies. Of course, it's necessary for us to tell our stories and to listen to the stories of others. This is the only way we have to understand and communicate our philosophies. Telling stories has become one of my favorite activities, and one of the most healing, helpful habits I have. Meditating on beautiful thoughts is surely my most joyful habit.

I have lived a full life with diabetes for more than 40 years. Professionally, I am an educator and author working in the fields of health, human behavior, and motivation. I feel that my life has been an experience demonstrating the healing power of spirituality. For that I am grateful. That is why I have earnestly sought to understand where and how to fit the spiritual component into health care, especially for people challenged by a chronic disease.

According to Dr. Rachel Naomi Remen, author of *Kitchen Table Wisdom*, "Everyone is a story." Over the past 24 years, I have shared my thoughts and stories with thousands of people throughout the United States, Canada, Australia, and Europe. The response I have consistently received (and the reward I cherish) is that people share their stories with me. I believe what Joseph Campbell said, "We shall come to the center of our own existence and, where we had thought to be alone, we shall be with all the world." When we are aware of our own stories, we can realize the power of being the author of the story.

Early on, I discovered the value of aphorisms— short statements with concentrated meaning. I agree with Southey's observation: "Be brief; for it is with words as with sunbeams—the more they are condensed, the deeper they burn." Reading aphorisms had the magical ability to call forth my stories, my philosophies, my meanings for life. I began collecting aphorisms, quotations, poetry, and stories when I was in grade school. I continue to this day. This book is full of them.

The purpose of this book is to help you find your meaning in your life experiences and to develop a philosophy that is both helpful and hopeful. Some of the aphorisms in this book are new to me, discovered as I researched this book. Other thoughts are old friends that have delighted, inspired, and comforted me for many years. May they connect you with your thoughts in ways that will lead you to strength, peace, and hope.

An old favorite by John W. Gardner is: "Some people strengthen the society just by being the kind of people they are." Those are the people whose stories I have shared in this book. My purpose in storytelling is to awaken your stories. Think of yourself as if you were a glass of soda with bubbles clinging to the sides of the glass and to the bottom. As you read this book, allow your stories to shake loose like those bubbles, rising to the surface of your mind where you can learn from them—and celebrate or discard them.

Ultimately, personal experience is the only valid means we have to understand life—past and present—and to make our choices for the future. Finding meaning in life requires a meditative style. I recommend meditative reading for this book. Robert Esbjornson, a retired religion professor from my alma mater, Gustavus Adolphus College, shared his definition of meditative reading with me.

Meditative reading is different from other kinds of reading. It is not reading to gather information, such as a cookbook when we are planning a meal. It is not reading for pleasure, such as a spy story, mystery, western, or romance. I read as if the author were addressing me and calling for a personal response . . . I read as if the author wanted to hear my personal reflections about not only the author's thoughts but my own life . . . I read expecting to find words that will illuminate and guide me to see things about myself and my situations . . . .

I am free from pressure to read so many pages per sitting, free from the need to comprehend the whole, free to respond to a phrase, sentence, or paragraph that strikes me as a message to me. Weeks may pass before I come to the end of the book.

Books for meditative reading may vary greatly. It is not the genre of a book that makes the difference; it is the manner in which we read it. Think of books as "angels" or messengers of God. Be hospitable when you read, as if you were entertaining an angel. Such reading is a great adventure! You never know when you will read something that will transform you!

Why do I, and I think you as well, need meditative reading? We are more than physical organisms . . . more than social animals . . . and more than minds interested in ideas and information. We also are souls. "Soul" is an aspect of ourselves that is hard to explain but that we experience in many situations and relationships. There is a hunger in us for what is beyond us, for what is complete, satisfying. It is hard to label this hunger, although the psalmists try when they write poetry about the thirst for God. Meditative reading is for ourselves as souls, not as social engineers and producers.

Two aphorisms come to mind.

What lies behind us and what lies before us are tiny matters compared to what lies within us.
– Oliver Wendell Holmes

The eyes believe themselves; the ears believe others; the heart believes the truth.
–Ibo proverb

Meditative reading is done with the heart—not the miraculously automatic muscle in the middle of the chest but the knowing in the center of our being. I ask each of you to read this book with your heart and, in so doing, to find your own meaning and personal application.

"Esbj" also encourages meditative listening as part of a meditative lifestyle.

Meditative listening opens us to messages we often miss in conversation. So often we hear the words but not the wisdom. Listen for something that touches your soul. It may be a familiar word used differently by the one speaking. It may be an emotional tone that signals a deep experience that has shaken the person. It may be something said by a person who you thought was always predictable that causes you to see that person in a new light. It may be a body language conveying a secret not readily shared in words.

Meditative reading, listening, and living give us insights into ourselves. These insights can lead to healing—if you give it time and your intention to heal. Several of the meditations in this book describe my son's injury as a baby and the years that it took for me to heal emotionally and spiritually. Give yourself time, but all the while remain a seeker of healing.

Now, clearly a chronic disease cannot be, in the conventional sense, healed, but it can be managed. Your insights can help you fit diabetes into a whole and healthy life, taking a holistic approach to living with it day to day. In turn, this can help you with the other aspect of diabetes—its long duration.

We usually measure time in cycles—days, weeks, months, seasons, years. Consider the seasons of your life as you read. What season are you experiencing outside, in nature right now? What season are you experiencing on the inside? Clearly, if nature sets us a good example, getting stuck in one season or another can't be nourishing over the long run. Observing the cycles of nature can give you wisdom for your own cycles.

For me, **Summer** is characterized by Joy and invites creativity and playfulness. We're on vacation. It helps to remind us of why we manage diabetes: so we can celebrate life. **Fall** brings the harvest of Wisdom from the stories and experiences we have collected for a lifetime. **Winter** comes so we can draw our energy in and rest. Winter's unique gift is in the fact that it requires us to have Courage, and our wintry experiences give us courage. **Spring** connects us with our Faith and leads to hope.

For all the seasons celebrated in this book, I have selected quotes or stories that I believe have universal application. These come from Jewish, Christian, and American Indian traditions as well as the centuries-old wisdom of people the world over. I have also included some personal reflections from my faith tradition of Christianity.

Whether or not you have a religion, you do have spiritual questions. I hope that sharing my personal stories will awaken in you an awareness of your own stories of faith.

When the American Diabetes Association asked me to write this book, they used one word to describe it: spiritual. I knew that two spiritual qualities would help me: humility and wisdom. With the first I would receive the second. I hope I have. Shall we begin?

The Seasons of the Spirit

The repetition in nature may not be a mere recurrence.
It may be a theatrical "encore."

–G.K. Chesterton

Together, let's read this quote meditatively. I will share my own understanding of it. Then, I invite you to read Chesterton's quote meditatively and record your thoughts about it in writing. When you just "think" your response, the insight can dissolve quickly. When you put it down in words, you remember it, you can come back and savor it, or you can hand it to someone else to enjoy. Written, it lasts longer.

I like the idea that it is my "Encore!" that brings the seasons of the spirit back on the stage again and again. My choice has brought about their return. Courage, Faith, Wisdom, and Joy do not automatically recur in my life. I choose to invite their powerful, yet peace-giving, presence. The words "theatrical encore" tell me that this is not a whisper. We shout ENCORE! There is neither timidity nor confusion. My desire for these spiritual values is utterly clear.

I call on Courage every moment of every day. Yes, I need courage in times of great challenges, but I also need courage to live each day according to my values and my convictions. Faith is the mysterious season. I need faith because we do not have all the answers. It waits in my soul for my quieted mind and turning within—my faith calls up Faith. I ask for Wisdom every day to make the choices that will give me a good quality of life. Wisdom guides my choice each time I shout ENCORE for Courage and Joy.

And Joy. I need Joy. I want Joy. ENCORE!

Summer

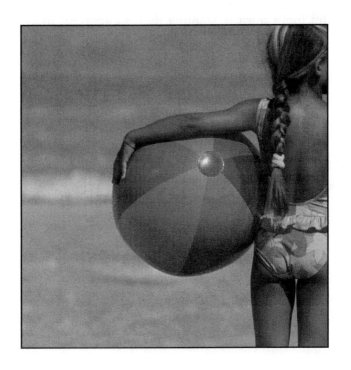

Introduction to Summer

Ah, what do your senses tell you about summer? Warm breezes gently stroking your face, the aroma of freshly mowed grass, the sound of birds greeting one another, the colorful parade of flowers in gardens and fields, and the taste of vine-ripened tomatoes and sweet corn. Summer. As grand as these outward signs of summer are, there is a playful inner spirit to summer that is important to us. Actually it is a way of healthy coping. This playful spirit moves us to explore the spiritual quality of joy.

Summer's overall theme is joy. From the very first page in this section, you are encouraged to reflect on the resources around you and within you that give you joy and keep you joyful. I believe that joy is the motivation and the energy behind diabetes self-management. Our willingness to engage in diabetes self-management is fueled by our desire to enjoy life.

Nature provides the stage for you to consider your environment and explore the lessons of the earth. Along with nature, we focus on the nurture we can receive from some of the great thinkers of all time. Voices that you hear include Helen Keller,

William Shakespeare, Ralph Waldo Emerson, the Bible, the Talmud, and a variety of poets and artists. A Kanem proverb from a twelfth century African civilization invites you to consider your own philosophy and reason for managing diabetes: "We will water the thorn for the sake of the rose."

From the seemingly fragile new beginnings of Spring to the fullness of Summer, we can reflect on the life cycle of flowers, ponder the metaphor of oak trees, and play with the thought that even a blade of grass has its own angel. Emerson said that "the earth laughs in flowers." Such thoughts can awaken you to the beauty and joy that surround you everyday—whether you're in a garden or a grocery store.

Along with joy and beauty, Summer also brings the power outages of summer storms and chores like mowing the lawn. Make some metaphors of your own. Power outages are the low blood sugars that can be prevented or treated. Mowing a lawn symbolizes the routine of life. I have to mow the lawn. I have to brush my teeth. I have to monitor blood glucose. I have to do some chores in life. I get to fly kites, hike, go on picnics, pick flowers—and experience playfulness, creativity, and Joy.

Summer is the time to explore music, laughter, beauty, and optimism. To think about joyful ways of supporting yourself and supporting others. Bring joy with you as you ponder the meditations in Summer.

Your success and happiness lie in you . . .
Resolve to keep happy, and your joy and you shall
form an invincible host against difficulties.
–Helen Keller

Today the summer spirit whisks us away like the wind playing with helium-filled balloons. The balloons had been held to the ground with lead weights. Those metaphoric "lead weights" are the heavy thoughts and concerns we all have.

What is currently weighing you down? With pen and paper handy, empty your head and your heart of all that concerns you at present. Write it down. Then, focus your attention on the spiritual wind that lifts your soul.

"Spiritual wind" can be a metaphor for the forces of light, joy, rejuvenation, faith, and hope. Now, take up your pen and fill your paper and your heart with everything you can think of that lifts your soul.

According to Dr. Rachel Naomi Remen, author of *Kitchen Table Wisdom*, the purpose of life is to grow in wisdom and to learn how to love better. She believes this can be accomplished through service to others.

Consider the ways you can be of service to those around you. For example, the simple act of holding the door for another person is a service. Have past experiences of service proved to be uplifting to you? List some of the possibilities for service today.

We used to have two huge, silver maple trees in our yard. After a particularly cold winter, one of them died. I was really stunned. The tree had seemed so healthy . . . and it had been part of our yard, almost like a member of our family.

We asked a tree specialist about the situation, and he said that silver maples have roots close to the surface. So, when there is a bitterly cold winter, the roots are affected by the cold. We decided to make a large ring around the remaining silver maple. The ring is bounded by large, round rocks and is filled with wood shavings, a blanket of insulation to protect the roots.

Nature had reinforced yet another important life lesson: Prevention. This lesson caused me to ask myself, "Am I doing as much for my own current and future health as I am for our tree?" I can meditate on that thought after a vigorous walk followed by a cooldown in the backyard. And, while cooling down, I look for lessons elsewhere.

And this our life . . . Finds tongues in trees, books in running brooks, Sermons in stones, and good in everything.
                                    –William Shakespeare

No pessimist ever discovered the secrets of the stars or sailed to an uncharted land or opened a new heaven to the human spirit.

–Helen Keller

Optimism is mostly a cherished attribute. Instinctively people understand that life is better when they can view it with hope rather than despair. Dr. Robert Schuller refers to optimism as "possibility thinking." From sociologists to historians to motivational speakers, we hear about the "can do" approach to life.

Optimism has built civilizations, negotiated unlikely peace treaties, started businesses, and discovered cures. In day-to-day living, it is optimism that means diabetes and joy can exist side by side in life . . . in each life affected by diabetes.

Some people seem to be naturally optimistic, but all of us have pessimism and cynicism knocking on the door . . . daily. The choice for all of us is to decide who we will let in the door—the door to our minds. Reflect on the thoughts that nourish your mind on a daily basis. Choose your mental nourishment as carefully as you choose physical nourishment.

A friend of mine shared a delightful way in which she helps herself regain a sense of control when her life is out of balance, stressed, or simply too busy. She walks into the family room of their home and looks at the shelf holding her collection of ducks. She reports: "I feel reassured and calm when I see that *somewhere* in my life . . . .

I have all my ducks in a row!"

Barbara Johnson carried a variation of that theme in her newsletter *The Love Line:* "When Life seems chaotic and you feel overwhelmed, take a deep breath, get your ducks in a row . . . and take 'em in the tub with you!"

Humor, a brief break, a new perspective . . . . You don't need a collection of ducks to tap into those stress managers. Consider how you utilize humor and a break to get a new perspective.

Support should never be viewed as something needed by weak people. Support is the reason that strong people are strong. We all need to feel supported.

Years ago, I heard former President Gerald Ford's son Steven make a presentation to 400 women in Minneapolis. His was a light-hearted speech on "Life in the White House" . . . when he was a teenager. He told us many funny stories, especially about his teenage perspective on having to include a secret service agent in all of his youthful activities!

In the middle of his talk, he suddenly stopped and said, "Before I forget, I want to say, 'Thank you'." He went on to share with us that his mother, Betty Ford, had had a mastectomy when he was a teenager. He knew that it had been a difficult experience for her. He asked her how she'd made it.

Betty told her son that she had made it because of cards, notes, and letters from women all over the United States who had written to tell her that they had had the same surgery. They had made it, and she was in their prayers.

Believing that at least one woman in the group may have written to his mother, he offered thanks to all of us. So, who needs support? The first lady of the United States of America . . . and each and every one of us.

After enlightenment, there's still the laundry.

–Chinese proverb

Being "in the moment" is not mysterious. Being in the moment is being aware of life, observing what is happening right now, and not thinking about last week or tomorrow. This is the only way to receive the messages of the moment. There are practical benefits to this practice as well as the celebrated rewards of peace and the appreciation of beauty. For example, as a practical benefit, we can see the impact of food and exercise on blood glucose levels by being in the moment.

Being in the moment also means that we notice the tiny buds on the trees as Spring's warmth encourages their appearance and then, the fullness of the leaves when Summer takes over Spring's task. Being in the moment as we talk with a friend or help a stranger helps us see love in action.

Being in the moment helps me keep my balance. I need to think beautiful thoughts to feed my soul, to encounter great wisdom to enlighten my mind, and to experience blood glucose results to guide my decisions. Life is lived in both the huge and small, the eloquent and the humble, the grand Aha's and the simple, necessary tasks.

Help me to balance beauty, wisdom, and duty.

Poetic language is powerful and far-reaching. In fact, truly great literature applies to us all.

I was studying Shakespeare in Europe in 1968 when Robert Kennedy and Martin Luther King, Jr., were assassinated. My sadness and shock were great, but I couldn't find language to express my feelings. Then I read *Measure for Measure* by William Shakespeare, and the following lines flew directly to my heart.

But man, proud man, dressed in a little brief authority plays such fantastic tricks before high heaven as makes the angels weep.

The image of angels weeping with me gave a context to my experience: A loss of such magnitude that the angels wept. This idea of a divine support group gave me strength and started my healing. I felt better because I had connected with words that gave meaning to my profound feelings. And I felt lifted up by angelic images more powerful than words.

Healing is necessary before we can find the required energy to manage diabetes and all the other life tasks before us. Be open to the many and, often unexpected, sources for healing.

Life is a university whose lessons encompass a wide array of subjects. If Life is the university, then Nature is surely one of its noblest, most honored professors.

I cherish the lessons that Nature teaches me and the process that leads to each lesson. Our experience with nature provides the insights that lead to the Aha!

The Mississippi River is nicknamed, the "Mighty Mississippi" for good reason. Strong current etches shorelines like an artist's paintbrush creates a picture. One day as I was enjoying the ever-changing view of the river's shoreline from a boat, I saw another aspect of the current. Although the boat's engines had been cut back, the boat was moving swiftly downstream.

Swift current increases fuel efficiency when one is going downstream. Likewise, the strong current makes an upstream trip more difficult, and much more fuel is consumed in the process.

Professor Nature raised its eyebrows in lovely, puffy, white clouds. The question posed to me was: As current is to the river, what are the outside forces in your life that help you get where you're going more efficiently, with less drain on your energy? What are the outside forces that make "headway" in diabetes or any life task more difficult?

A professor of Classics wrote in an essay that the word "yes" is the most powerful word in the English language. I was immediately reminded of a trip that Robert Fulghum made to Minneapolis in 1990. Fulghum, a popular author, made it known that he had a fantasy about conducting an orchestra. The marketing director of the Minneapolis Chamber Symphony wrote him and offered her orchestra.

He accepted the invitation to come to Minneapolis. But, shortly after doing so, he learned of serious political and financial difficulties within the Chamber Symphony. As he flew to Minneapolis, he wondered if any musicians would be there to play.

When he arrived, the stage was full of musicians. Fulghum said, "The fact that there are musicians on stage means the 'Yes!' goes on."

Reflect on the experiences in your life when you have been carried by the "Yes" or you have chosen "Yes." Consider a situation you are facing today. What does it mean to choose "Yes"?

Earth laughs in flowers.

–Ralph Waldo Emerson

Smile whenever you see flowers erupting from the ground. What is it that caused the earth to laugh there?

Were the daffodils a response to a gentle tickling created by a rake?

Did the tulips emerge when rain trickled down and the earth chuckled in delight?

Is the earth's floral laughter its way to express joy and gratitude to its creator?

I want to think so. I am inspired by this thought. I wonder how it is that I am expressing my joy and gratitude?

May my life be my "thank you."

A faithful friend is the medicine of life.
                                    —Ecclesiastes 6:16

The notion that an apple a day keeps us healthy has given way to the results of research demonstrating the power and importance of social support: we need friends.

Giving friendship may be even more health-promoting than being on the receiving end of friendship. Dr. Hans Selye, a Montreal physician who was considered an expert in stress management, reported that giving of himself to help others was the single greatest stress reducer in his life.

To receive the "medicine" of friendship, give friendship. As is said about love, the more you give, the more you receive.

Help me to be a faithful friend.

Some of the scariest storms I have experienced have been in the summer . . . especially the storms at night. The crashing thunder and awesome lightning make me feel insignificant in comparison. Strong wind is especially frightening at night because I can't see what it's doing.

I can remember having to go out one night in such a storm to check on the rainspouts to make sure they were attached, to carry the water from the eaves away from the house. A gust of wind nearly knocked me over. I found my way to our oak tree and grabbed hold to steady myself. As I regained my balance, I felt a surge of comfort and security, a gift from the large, solid oak tree.

We all encounter storms in our lives. Diabetes can be considered one of them. Each of us needs to find our own tree. Hold on to it. Receive its support. Its many branches can include family, friends, church and synagogue, the American Diabetes Association, the heroes and heroines of life past and present.

At a party one evening, I overheard my husband telling someone: "The best thing that ever happened to me was marrying someone with diabetes. We live such a healthy life." He is my oak. Reflect on yours.

If rewards were not important, I doubt that there would be trophies for athletic achievement, gold stars on the music sheets of piano students, or corporate achievement awards for departments and individuals.

Rewards can be external "things," like trophies or trinkets. Or rewards can be inner messages to ourselves that celebrate the success of a job well done, providing polish to our self-image. Most of us look forward to some kind of a reward for our efforts.

As part of a lecture I routinely gave in a diabetes program in the 1970s, I made the observation that there was an odd sort of reward system in diabetes management. It seemed to be: If you take really good care of yourself, maybe in 15 or 20 years, you won't go blind. Negative half-promises far out in the future are unlikely rewards for today's behavior.

To influence today's behavior, you need a short-term reward, if not right away, then soon. Receiving a reward is the boost that many of us need to keep working on behaviors like regular exercise, consistent blood glucose monitoring, and healthful eating.

Rewards are important. What rewards do you respond to most positively?

Sometimes I need inspiration from great, thunderous, amazing, and magnificent music. Whether orchestral or vocal, the music floods me with its power and lifts me above the world that causes distress.

Sometimes I need quiet inspiration, the kind that comes as I sit on a dock at sunset watching a distant city skyscape or the forest's tree-lined contour.

And then, I am amazed by the silence . . . the quiet around me allowing the music within me to be heard.

**Help me, this day,
to hear the music of my soul.**

A merry heart doeth good like a medicine.

–Proverbs 17:22

If King Solomon had written a book on the effects of humor on health, he might have called it "Amusing Grace." Surely, it is humor that warms us and strengthens us.

Some people feel in control over anything they can laugh at or about. The following story was shared with me as an example of being in control of an otherwise difficult situation.

A woman who'd had both legs amputated below the knee left her prostheses in a changing room at the club when she exercised in the swimming pool. Because the door left eighteen inches or so open to the floor, people could see two legs, and some wondered if a woman in the changing room were in need of help. To deal with the curious and the concerned, she put a sign on the door: "My legs are resting. I'm in the pool."

Joy is not in things; it is in us.

–Richard Wagner

Famous people often get asked for advice, formulas for success, or descriptions of their personal happiness. The English poet, John Keats, offered this:

> *Give me books, fruit, French wine, and fine weather, and a little music out of doors, played by someone I do not know.*

If you suddenly found yourself "famous," how would you respond to a journalist who asked you the question: "What is it in life that makes you happy?"

Then, how would you respond to the question: "What is your source of joy?"

Comedian David Letterman remarked once that he was struck by the wording on a bag he saw in a hardware store: "Worm and Grub Killer." Letterman said that if we named products based on outcomes, then "candy bars" really should be called "fat-boy zit bars." Whereas a "juicy steak" may sound appealing, "blubber" and "lard" usually don't.

Finish the following descriptions à la Letterman:

rich desserts would be_____

high-fat meats would be_____

high-salt, high-fat snacks would be_____

fast food would be_____

After smiling about our creative responses, we might even feel like making healthier choices.

When blood sugar gets low, quite commonly a person's disposition sours. One day when my son was about seven years old, he noticed that I was "out of sorts." He looked at me intently and said: "Are ya low, Mom?" His innocent question startled me into perspective. I said to him: "No, I'm not low. I was just being crabby . . . and I'm sorry."

That experience became a source of humor for our family as we gave exaggerated versions of the question: "Are ya low, Mom?" The story became a way to balance as we all came to realize the value of chilling out when any of us was under stress. We learned to respect one another's space and individual needs for regaining perspective.

When an occasionally grumpy little boy got off the school bus, I gave him time and space.

Everyone needs that, not just people with diabetes.

Some people regard discipline as a chore. For me, it is a kind of order that sets me free to fly.

–Julie Andrews

There have to be times when the disciplined life of diabetes self-management seems like a chore. But, can it also be a structure that allows for greater freedom?

With the discipline of a well-planned series of meals, extra food, and blood glucose monitoring materials, people can bring diabetes on canoe trips, climbing expeditions, vacations, and all the day-to-day activities that include work as well as play.

Diabetes can even accompany us on spontaneous excursions. Prior planning sets the scene for spontaneity. Extra food in the glove box of the car, a book bag, briefcase, or purse can supply the fuel for a flight of fantasy. If your blood glucose meter is a daily companion, a safe landing is likely to result.

Set yourself free to fly.

Every blade of grass has its Angel that bends over it and whispers, "Grow, grow."

–The Talmud

Some people see angels as winged, ethereal creatures playing golden harps. Others think of angels as being invisible but with a very real presence in their lives. Still others give angelic qualities to the people in their lives who seem to "be there" whenever help is needed with a pot of soup, a shoveled walk, or a cheery phone call. In all cases, angels are the forces of good.

Reflect on the "angels"—visible and invisible—in your life who have encouraged your growth and healing.

Thank them.

Meditating on the words on the previous page can bring some questions to the surface. Do we always recognize angels?

Is it possible that people who annoy us are actually angels? Some of the annoyance that many of us experience with people in relation to our diabetes, is that they "nag" us. "Are you testing?" asks a parent. "Should you be eating that?" asks a spouse, coworker, or friend. "How's the weight?" asks a health care professional.

It's time to ask ourselves: "Are they nagging me or are they genuinely concerned and just asking me how I'm doing?"

Is it possible that their questions are motivated by their love and their desire to see us do well and be well? To grow, grow.

Maybe they don't fully recognize who we are. Are you a rebel? Or are you a responsible person making the best choices you can?

Maybe we all need to talk more.

Summer is a good time to store up visual images of natural beauty that can be used throughout the winter for visualization exercises. (This is especially true for those of us from the north!)

Mary Casey, chaplain at Fairview University Medical Center in Minneapolis, combines breathing and mental imagery in the meditations she shares with patients. According to Mary, when we focus on our breathing, we let go of distracting thoughts. To open ourselves to God's healing messages, it can be helpful to focus on an image that is peace-giving. Many people choose a setting by a lake or river.

Mary invites people to imagine the waves of the lake bringing in any anxiety from the center of the lake to the shoreline where God's arms will receive it. The wave is then sent back out cleansed. God's arms are much like the shore of the lake, able to receive and hold anything brought to it. Mary refers to this image as a "place of grace," and as we "lean into it," we can hear God's gentle voice saying the beautiful words:

Be still and know that I am God
Be still and know that I am
Be still and know that I
Be still and know that
Be still and know
Be still and
Be still
Be

Oh that I had wings like a dove! I would fly away and be at rest; yea, I would wander afar, I would lodge in the wilderness.

–Psalm 55:6–7

Do you know where to go for a good dose of the Summer Spirit whenever you need it? My neighbor Mary has long ago moved away, but her legacy remains as a gift of summer when I need it.

Mary used to plant daffodils in the woods behind her house . . . not in a row, but at random. Always, it was a delightful surprise to spot them. She called me one day and said simply, "What a wonderful day to be a daffodil."

My imagination did the rest. I pictured myself as a daffodil gently bobbing in the breeze. Stress was gone. I smiled all day whenever I thought about being a daffodil protected by the surrounding woods, gently kissed by streaks of sunlight, and tickled by gentle winds.

Help me to be a breath of summer in the lives of people around me.

Look for the rainbow, that gracious thing, made up of tears and light.

–Samuel Taylor Coleridge

We see rainbows when there has been rain. It is a natural phenomenon caused by the combination of rain and sunshine. The rainbow was God's promise to Noah and future generations that never again would the entire earth be covered with water. The flood that covered the whole earth and caused Noah to build the ark and save pairs of animals would not recur.

But, God did not promise an end to rain. Indeed, the earth cannot survive if we do not receive rain on a regular and restorative basis. So it is with our lives.

No one can promise us an end to our tears. But the rainbow reminds us that life will not be only tears. We will experience light—as laughter, as love, as joy, as renewed hope. The rainbow also reminds us that we cannot have only light. We need both sunshine and rain, joy and tears . . . for it is their combination that produces beauty and beams a promise.

The rainbow's beauty is today's pleasure and tomorrow's promise that there is always hope.

The river is a wonderful book with a new story to tell everyday.
–Mark Twain

Life provides many classrooms—from libraries and schools to rivers and mountains. The river is my favorite classroom.

Whether the river takes us to towns, festivals, or fishing, there are stories to hear at every bend. But, when we are very still and watch the river and listen carefully, we hear our own stories . . . welling up from the river within us.

The river has taught me to listen; you will learn from it, too. The river knows everything; one can learn everything from it.
–Hermann Hesse

Meditations on Diabetes

Prevention is a very important part of diabetes self-care. We want to prevent the complications of diabetes. But prevention is not the whole picture. Can you imagine getting out of bed in the morning, stretching, and saying: "Well, another day to prevent blindness"?

Beyond prevention of early death, disability, and disease, there is the promotion of life, health, and well-being. The reason we eat nutritiously, take medication (if prescribed), exercise, and monitor blood glucose is so that we can enjoy life.

We will water the thorn for the sake of the rose.
                                        –Kanem proverb

Zig Ziglar, a motivational expert, compares motivation to a fire in a fireplace. When the fire ceases to burn, you take a poker, poke the logs a few times, and soon have a roaring blaze again. In poking the logs, the movement of air creates a partial vacuum in the fireplace. Since nature abhors a vacuum, fresh air rushes in to fill the space, bringing the additional oxygen that ignites the smoldering logs and . . . you have a fire!

According to Ziglar's analogy, people are like those logs. Internally there is a smoldering fire, and often all we need is a little stoking from some outside force to get our fire going again.

We need "pokers" to rekindle our inner fire.

Who, what, where are the pokers in your life?

A sign at a summer camp said: GREAT WALK. I had been told that the path was indeed a great walk, both for the natural wonders of plants, flowers, trees, ponds, and resident animals as well as for the rigor of the physical workout. I reflected on the sign and thought of its deeper meaning in my life's walk.

Just as rain gear helps me enjoy the sight of a raindrop splashing off a glistening leaf, so does the "rain gear" of blood glucose meter and carbohydrates help me engage more fully in life.

If Life is to be a great walk, then our knapsack must be packed with all that we will need physically, mentally, and spiritually: granola bars to feed your body, books to fuel your mind, and experiences that your soul uses to nourish your heart.

**Shoulder your pack and take your walk.
And listen.**

The state of Victoria in Australia is greatly committed to promoting health. Car races are sponsored by Vic Health Promotion. Cigarettes are heavily taxed, and the taxes support health promotion.

The billboards are wonderful. They advertise exercise and lifelong, healthy activity. They show active children, adolescents, young adults, adults, and seniors. The message is one of health and self. Health cannot just "happen." Health is a direct result of choices we make.

What billboards do you see in your neighborhood, on your way to work, or driving other places? What are they promoting? What is the message?

Most importantly, what are the "billboards" in your mind? What are the messages you choose (or allow) on display in your mind?

Good quality of life is the ultimate outcome that each of us seeks. The definition of quality depends on individual goals, needs, and values.

Reflect on what quality of life means to you. This is the foundation of your motivation, the reason that you are willing to manage diabetes on a day-to-day, hour-by-hour basis.

People report the following definitions of quality of life:

- feeling well so that I can enjoy family life
- being able to participate in all areas of life with energy
- being free of complications of diabetes
- immersing myself in life in spite of complications
- having physical and mental energy and spiritual peace

Over the next several pages, we consider a process that is one way to achieve a better quality of life.

Ask yourself **questions**. If life is a journey, then it is a question that begins it and questions that cause us to continue the journey. What does quality of life mean to you? Continue the quest.

Uplift yourself and others. This will energize you spiritually.

In the 1970s, I met a woman from rural Minnesota. She knew that I had diabetes. She came up and said one sentence to me: "I just want you to know that I have had diabetes for 44 years."

I drank her in! She looked perfectly healthy. At that point I had had diabetes for 17 years and played the "game" that many of us play . . . trying to project what my future health would be. Because no one can know the future, I found it enormously uplifting to meet this woman. She was living "proof" that some people live very well with diabetes. I was inspired.

More than 20 years later, I was at the club where my family and I work out. I noticed a young woman in her 20s using a blood glucose meter in the locker room. I commented: "I have one of those, too."

She looked at me and said: "I have only recently been diagnosed."

I responded with that powerful sentence: "I've had diabetes for 41 years."

She exclaimed: "Oh, that's so encouraging!"

"I know," I said. "That's why I told you."

Adapt to the ongoing changes in life. Adaptability may be our single greatest ability. According to Dr. George Vaillant, a psychiatrist, "Stress does not kill us so much as ingenious adaptation to stress facilitates our survival."

From the *Criteria for Emotional Maturity* by Dr. William Menninger of the famed Menninger Clinic and Foundation comes a description that helps to define adaptability as "the ability to deal constructively with reality."

Applying that to diabetes means that we don't have to like having diabetes. But, if we are to have quality of life, then we need to adapt to what is and deal constructively with the reality of having diabetes.

What helps you to adapt? Blood glucose monitoring? Education programs? Your health care team? Family, friends, coworkers? Your spirit?

Listen to your inner wisdom. Your health care team can give you essential information for managing diabetes, but only you can know what is essential for managing your life.

Listen to your own values, goals, and needs. Connect with all the resources you have to live according to your values. Meet your needs as only you can. Set your own goals. The goals you set are the only ones you will have the energy to pursue and achieve.

Listen to yourself.

Integrate diabetes and life. Diabetes affects and is affected by all aspects of life. Empowerment is a process whereby we identify our goals and our problems and our resources. If quality of life (as defined by the individual) is the goal, and diabetes is the problem, then we identify all the external and inner resources to achieve our goals and overcome our problems. The outcome of this empowerment process is the integration of diabetes and life.

Diabetes cannot be left on the kitchen counter when we go shopping . . . or in the glove box when we pull into the employee parking lot . . . or in the bathroom when we leave on vacation.

Diabetes and life need to be integrated, so that diabetes gets managed and life gets enjoyed.

Teach all of your supporters how they can support you. Friends need to understand why timing of meals is important when we use insulin. Family members need to understand what's going on with blood glucose if we are to receive their cooperation. Our health care team needs to know who we are and what we value if we are to truly form an effective team.

People cannot read our minds. Share, communicate, . . . teach.

Yes! Keep looking for everything that is YES around you and within you. Connect with all the stories, people, and experiences that ignite your spirit and affirm what you value about life. Seek quality. Build a quality life.

Question

Uplift

Adapt

Listen

Integrate

Teach

Yes!

Mental visualization is a powerful tool for attaining goals. Psychologists tell us that we move in the direction of our most dominant thought. Another spin on that idea is to say that "expectation becomes self-fulfilling prophecy." We expect something to happen. We visualize the outcome. We move in that direction because we have transformed the goal into a blueprint.

There is one more important dimension of reaching a goal through visualization—belief. We must believe what we can only see in our mind's eye.

I shared this concept of mental imagery once with a bank president. He said he planned to use it in his golf game. Some weeks later I gave a program for his employees. When I saw him, I asked about his golf game. He reported that visualization had not worked for him. However, after my presentation he exclaimed to me, "That's it! I visualized, but I didn't believe. I'd say to myself, 'That's where I want the ball to go, but it won't.' I visualized but didn't believe."

Visualize and believe.

God made the sea, we make the ship; He made the wind, we make a sail; He made the calm, we make the oars.

—Senegal proverb

When people are able to move beyond the anger and denial that are quite natural responses to the diagnosis of diabetes, they stop placing blame and look within themselves for the strength and resources to live well with this challenge.

As is eloquently expressed in the Senegal proverb, we have a role to play, a responsibility, and an opportunity. The following affirmations come to mind as I meditatively read the Senegal proverb.

I have the responsibility for my life.
I have a blood glucose monitor; I will use it and act on the information.
I have a knowledgeable, caring health care team; I will see them regularly.
I have walking shoes; I will walk.

Help me to work with you.

Just trust yourself, then you will know how to live.
                              –Johann Wolfgang von Goethe

Distraction is a helpful technique for pain management. Many have reported that a toothache has virtually disappeared when the mind is distracted by a game, movie, or stimulating conversation. What is true for physical pain can also be true for mental and spiritual pain.

Make a list of distractions:

- a novel that literally takes you away to another place and time
- a movie that pulls you into its story from beginning to end
- a telephone call or visit with someone who cares about you
- a project in your house
- a visit to the library to explore its offerings
- a walk down the main street of a neighboring city
- meeting a friend for coffee in a new or favorite coffee shop

Go on with your own list, then tape it to the inside of a cupboard door in your kitchen. When your summer spirit fizzles, go to your list for refreshment.

A man's capacity is the same as his breadth of vision.

—Arab proverb

Graduations, confirmations, baptisms, and bar mitzvahs—all of these signs of "passage" bring me to a card shop. And once again, I ponder the questions these cards raise and apply them to my own life.

When I read the hopeful wishes for graduates about who they will become, I ask myself who I have become. With the help of the poetry and lofty phrases on the cards, I review my own life.

Will you be ethical? Wise? Honest? Compassionate? Will you be smart so that you can make your way in this world? Will you give more than you take? What will you value above all else? Who will remember you? Why?

The same integrity that guides our direction at work, in our homes, and with our friends is the personal integrity that guides our choices in managing diabetes.

Integrity is a wholeness of the spirit that causes our whole life to be in agreement. Integrity occurs when what we say and what we do are the same.

Beauty is not caused. It is.

                                    –Emily Dickinson

Apply that thought to joy. Joy is different from happiness, which can be caused. The causes for happiness are as many and as varied as there are people. We can be made happy because the weather is beautiful on a day we have planned a picnic or a bike ride. Happiness can be caused by an unending list of external factors that combine to provide us with what we think we want. While happiness is caused by outside circumstances, joy is a spiritual, inner quality.

> *While with an eye made quiet by the power of harmony, and the deep power of joy, we see into the life of things.*
>   –William Wordsworth

There are two thoughts from ancient scripture that shed insight into the source of joy and a means of tapping that source.

> *The Lord reigneth; let the earth rejoice.*
>   –Psalm 97:1

Serve the Lord with gladness; come before his presence with singing.

–Psalm 100:2

Consider what those two passages mean to you. Meditate on the joy in your life. What is its source? How do you access joy? Does your joy help you to "see into the life of things?"

A counselor told the story of meeting with a man whose life was totally out of control. His story included drugs, jail, and divorce. His body posture communicated his hopelessness.

The counselor said to him: "I see a boat being controlled by the swift current in the river. Wherever the current takes it, the boat goes. There are piles of jagged rocks in the river. The boat could crash."

The man quietly responded, "I see what you're saying."

"Look in the bottom of the boat," said the counselor. "What do you see?"

"Oars," was the man's response.

My blood glucose monitor and strips are the oars that I use to steer through the river of diabetes.

Thank you for the technology that helps me to stay healthy. Help me to use it.

That is happiness; to be dissolved into something completely great.

                              –Willa Cather

A blessing that diabetes has provided me is the opportunity to meet many wonderful people who are affected by diabetes either because they have it, a loved one has it, or they are health care professionals. Together we have worked on raising funds for research and supporting the programs of the American Diabetes Association.

We have helped one another to grow, to heal, to laugh again. We have rallied around people newly diagnosed with diabetes. We have been the community activists to get political support for diabetes education and supplies. We have helped to inform the broader community about diabetes.

We have moved outside of ourselves and our worlds to dissolve into the larger concern for others.

Table graces are said by many people and represent a wide diversity of religious and cultural traditions. Most of them express gratitude for food about to be received as well as an acknowledgement of our role in giving back as we have received. As we are nourished, may we so nourish life.

A table grace has long been part of a family tradition for me. Some years after I was diagnosed with diabetes, I received a new insight from our table grace. When I focus on my gratitude for the food and my responsibility of returned service, eating has a new meaning. I don't eat because I have to meet my insulin. I don't eat just because I'm hungry or the food tastes good. I eat as part of my service to life.

**Bless this food to our use and us
to Thy service.**

Be glad of life because it gives you the chance to love and to work and to play and to look at the stars.

–Henry Van Dyke

It is precisely because I am glad of life that I work at managing diabetes. Being "glad of life" can show itself in many ways. Basically, I see it as loving life itself. I experience this love standing in a field looking at the wildflowers, listening to the laughter of a small child, walking through my neighborhood appreciating with profound gratitude that I can walk . . . and I experience the gladness of life every morning when I awaken. "Thank you" are usually the first words I say.

I am reminded of the very first prayer our son said:

"Thank you, God, another day!"

To see a World in a Grain of Sand
And a Heaven in a Wild Flower
Hold Infinity in the palm of your hand
And Eternity in an hour . . .

–William Blake

One need not be a poet to see the infinite in the finite. Look around you today. See the beauty in a flower, then go beyond simple beauty, and see the divine. It's there. Open yourself to see, to hear, to smell, to feel, to be.

*Let no one ever come to you without leaving
better and happier. Be the living expression of
God's kindness; kindness in your face, kindness
in your eyes, kindness in your smile.*

–Mother Teresa

Sometimes we tell ourselves that we have nothing to give. The twinkling lights in the house across the street serve as a reminder that other people have and do and give. It's the yearning to give that creates our anguish. Human potential is at its greatest when we are able to give to help others.

We have lost Mother Teresa, but her loving, giving spirit will never die. That's what she was, "The living expression of God's kindness." Her legacy and her mandate is that we can all give. We have plenty.

Our brightest blazes of gladness are commonly kindled by unexpected sparks.

–Samuel Johnson

Summer symbolizes Joy. You can choose to have a Summer, Fall, Winter, or Spring moment whenever you need or desire them. They are moments of and experiences with Joy, Wisdom, Courage, and Hope.

To connect with a summer moment, you might engage in a mental-imagery activity. Sit in a comfortable chair in a quiet room where you are reasonably assured of not being disturbed. Quiet yourself. Close your eyes and focus on your breathing. Place your hand on your abdomen and feel your abdomen move as you breathe deeply.

When you begin to feel relaxed, travel in your mind's eye to a favorite summer place . . . a lake cabin, a bonfire on a beach, a backyard gazebo, a porch, or a park. Experience this cherished place with all of your senses. What do you see? What do you hear? What do you feel? What do you smell? What do you taste? Relax and savor this moment. When you want to return to the present, you just open your eyes.

Likewise you can return to your special seasonal moments whenever you need them. And celebrate them when they come spontaneously to you. The aroma of a fire, the sounds of a guitar or harmonica, a gentle breeze touching your face . . . any of these "reminders" can return you to your special place.

Be open to the lovely seasonal moments that "find" you unexpectedly.

There are some people who have the quality of richness and joy in them and they communicate it to everything they touch. It is first of all a physical quality; then it is a quality of the spirit.

–Thomas Wolfe

I need those people in my life. Their spirit ignites mine.

Reflect on the people you know who have the quality that Wolfe describes. They are refreshment for our souls as surely as water quenches our thirst.

My friend Anne has that quality of richness and joy. Every time I see her (most often by chance in the grocery store), her face lights up with warmth and joy and love. That quality was not extinguished after her sister died. Nor after her mother died. Nor after her cancer surgery. This quality is not physical. It is a quality of the spirit.

I am blessed that she has touched my life.

Friendship needs no words—it is solitude
delivered from the anguish of loneliness.

—Dag Hammarskjold

How do you differentiate between solitude and loneliness?

Loneliness can happen even when you're with other people. What are the elements that create loneliness? Is it a problem with people and situations outside of you? Or is loneliness created from a hurt deep inside you? Reflect on these questions. Go where they lead you.

Then, reflect on solitude. Can you be all alone and experience solitude but not loneliness? Does solitude mean that you have friends you could call or see . . . or friendships so deep that you're together in spirit even when you're physically separated?

Reflect on your friendships. Do they deliver you from loneliness and give you solitude? Think about how that happens.

Affirmation of life is the spiritual act by which man ceases to live unreflectively and begins to devote himself to his life with reverence in order to raise it to its true value. To affirm life is to deepen, to make more inward, and to exalt the will to live.

–Albert Schweitzer

I have based my work on the belief in three driving principles: Cope, Support, and Hope—the psychosocial/spiritual. In the mid-1980s, I wrote the following affirmations to accompany the seminar that I developed and still facilitate.

I will meet Life's challenges with a spirit of determination.

I will cope with Life's stresses, controlling what I can, and letting go of worry over stresses that I cannot control.

I will seek support whenever I need it. I will receive support gratefully and give it generously.

I will live Today well, remembering the lessons and happiness of Yesterday, and believing in the promises and hope of Tomorrow.

For today well-lived makes every yesterday a dream of happiness and every tomorrow a vision of Hope.

–Kalidasa

Fall

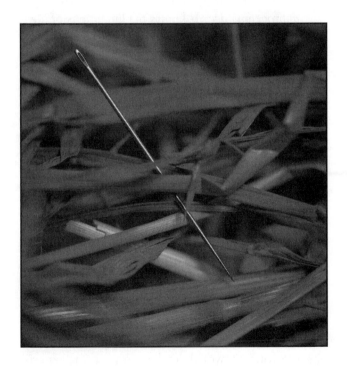

Introduction to Fall

I like spring, but it is too young. I like summer,
but it is too proud. So I like best of all autumn;
because its leaves are a little yellow, its tone
mellower, its colors richer. And it is tinged a little
with sorrow. Its golden richness speaks not of the
innocence of spring, nor of the power of summer,
but of the mellowness and kindly wisdom of
approaching age. It knows the limitations of life
and is content.

–Lin Yutang

This section explores among the falling leaves and seeks to uncover wisdom. Because school traditionally begins in the Fall, I see all of us riding the school bus of life to the classroom of our hearts. Come wholeheartedly into Fall. Reconnect with the wisdom you already have, the wisdom that has always been and always will be inside of you. Different from knowledge that changes with each new piece of information, wisdom is lasting and universal truth. Wisdom is profound and changeless.

Fall is the time to harvest and reflect on the wisdom found in family stories, African proverbs, your own ever-developing philosophy of life, observations of world leaders, and your experiences with life. You might, consider what Nobel Prize winner George Minot's "art of courageous living" means to you. Ask yourself about your expectations of life—do you expect guarantees?

As you reflect on your own experiences, consider how other people cope with a wide variety of life challenges. Viktor Frankl survived a Nazi concentration camp by choosing to help those around him. His profound insights can find application in our lives. Ancient Chinese medicine encourages being in the moment. Coupled with Goethe's wisdom that at each moment Nature reaches her goal, we are invited to see each moment as its own destination. We are not to worry about the coming winter. The work we do in the Fall—storing up wisdom—will feed us through the winters of our souls.

I encourage you to keep Wisdom as a traveling companion throughout your journey in life. Like the conductor of a great symphony orchestra, Wisdom brings into play at all the appropriate times, not the woodwinds or brass, but Courage, Faith, and Joy.

Knowledge is proud that he has learned so much;
Wisdom is humble that he knows no more.
                                        —William Cowper

Knowledge about diabetes has changed and continues to change. Years ago, we were told to soak our feet every day in water to which we added soap. Now we are told that daily soaking breaks down tissue, and soap is too drying. In other words, the new advice is: Dont soak your feet! Recommendations about insulin have changed from multiple injections (when we only had regular) to one shot (when intermediate-acting insulin was discovered) back to multiple injections following the Diabetes Control and Complications Trial (DCCT).

As knowledge changes, wisdom keeps our minds open to new information and the ongoing changes in therapies and lifestyle recommendations. Without this wisdom, we may view change as a frustrating betrayal of our trust in medicine and health care professionals. Wisdom kindly grants a fresh perspective and helps us accept change.

Thank you for wisdom.

I love the Fall of the year! Crisp air, leaves aflame in color waving from the trees, and excited children heading back to school.

As I watch the children walk toward the school bus for the first day of school, I see their smiles and hear the excited anticipation in their greetings. Their book bags will be full this afternoon when they get off the bus. Now they hold only shiny new crayons with a waxy aroma and blank notebooks awaiting the touch of young fingers and explorations of eager minds.

I realize that I envy the children. Life is new again each Fall. Then I receive an insight. Fall can continue to be a new beginning, even now. In fact, each day I ride the school bus of life to the classroom of my heart.

My English lesson can come, from any of the books on my shelf . . . the ones I've been meaning to read. History exists in every building I visit, every person I meet. My education is not limited to the traditional subjects. Diabetes has been an important teacher since I was diagnosed in 1957. I continue to learn about life and health, coping with challenges, giving of myself to help others, experiencing spiritual places, and receiving the grace and love I find there.

So, again today, I board the school bus of life and eagerly anticipate the lessons I will surely receive.

Dr. Clarissa Pinkola Estes, author of *Women Who Run with the Wolves* and *The Gift of Story* refers to stories as medicine. She notes that "Tales, legends, myths, and folklore are learned, developed, numbered, and preserved the way a pharmacopoeia is kept. A collection of cultural stories, and especially family stories, is considered as necessary for long and strong life as decent food, decent relationships, and decent work." She informs us that in her family the telling of stories is an essential spiritual practice.

What are the stories you have heard around the kitchen or dining room table? What do you know about yourself based on family stories? What strengths have people in your family shown through their life stories? Many families have "horror" stories. What are your family's "healing" stories? Tell them. Again and again.

**Help me that my life
can be a healing story for all to read.**

Throughout our lives we develop a philosophy (or a series of them). One purpose I have in writing this book is to encourage readers to become aware of and develop a helpful philosophy, one that will give meaning to their lives and help them live comfortably with their experiences.

Philosophy can seem obscure at times, but its value is in getting us to think. Consider the following story and reflect on the meaning it holds for you.

A familiar philosophy is found in the adage: "If Life gives you lemons, make lemonade. Do the best with what you've been given. I have found that philosophy useful at times, but trite and irritating at other times in my life. I received a great insight into my personal philosophy when I heard a Lutheran pastor say from the pulpit: "If life gives you lemons and you don't like lemonade, then throw the lemons back and demand strawberries!"

The original philosophy was missing the important element of choice. If I don't like lemonade, I don't have to make it. We do have choices.

Support is an important part of life and, certainly, an important part of living well with the challenges of diabetes. In an ideal world, everyone with whom we interact would understand diabetes and willingly support us . . . in the manner we prefer.

But the world is not ideal. We may find some supportive people in our lives but not as many as we would like. There are three important elements involved in getting the support that we need and want.

1) We need to be clear in our understanding of how we want to be supported and clearly communicate our needs to the appropriate people.

Are any of these ways that you would like to get support?

- families would join us in healthy eating and regular exercise
- friends would live healthy lifestyles, too
- insurance companies would provide all that we need
- employers would be flexible and non-discriminatory
- health care providers would be knowledgeable and willing to help

2) All of our would-be supporters need to know us.

Those who would rightly understand someone must first read the whole story.

–Proverb

And, if they don't "read" our story, we need to read it to them.

3) We need to actively support the people whom we would like to support us. Support is a circle. The giving and the receiving blend into one. The reward in giving support was described by Abraham Lincoln:

To ease another's heartache is to forget one's own.

At a diabetes conference, Dr. Jean Philippe Assal of the University of Geneva, Switzerland, showed a slide of a lovely pastoral scene. But, it had a big blob in the middle, almost as if a drop of paint had fallen on the canvas by mistake. He said: "Diabetes is a rupture on the landscape of peoples lives." Dr. Assals comment was a compassionate recognition of the impact that diabetes has in the lives of people. He was speaking to physicians and reaching them with an important message about the human implication of diabetes.

I listened reflectively—appreciating that his message was reaching physicians and, at the same time, responding to his words from my perspective as a person who has diabetes.

What does a rupture mean? Does that mean we are to cover it up and hide it? Ignore it and pretend it's not there? Or, is it possible that this rupture on the landscape of our lives can become a distinctive part of its beauty?

When I left home, my mother sent me a poem that, for me, answers this question.

The rift in the chest of a mountain,
The twist in the trunk of a tree,
The water-cut cave in the hollow,
The rough, rocky rim of the sea . . .

Each one has a scar of distortion,
Yet each has this sermon to sing,
"The presence of what would deface me,
Has made me a beautiful thing."

—Anonymous

Consider the ways in which diabetes can make your spirit beautiful.

Words can release stress and restore feelings of peace. How? By promoting mental images that relax and rejuvenate us.

FLOAT is a word that reminds me to relax. I think about being in the water at the beach, facing large waves, and choosing not to struggle but, instead, to float. I see a feather or a leaf gently floating through the air. Both the feather and the leaf whisper their healing message and timeless wisdom: Float.

We know that mental images are powerful tools in stress management. But just when we need them the most, when we are under the greatest stress, we find it difficult to get the soothing image on the projection screen of our minds. That's why words are so helpful. Can you say the word "elephant" without seeing one?

Identify the words that bring healing, restorative images. Say them.

Life's lessons are everywhere, her wisdom is ever available. In my first experience with snorkeling, I learned two of life's lessons—one philosophical, one practical.

It was a windy day, and the water was choppy. With my snorkeling mask in place, I could look at the surface disturbance and then look down below the surface and see where the watery world was calm, the beauty untouched by surface winds. I immediately connected with the idea that surface irritations in life can distract us from the deeper issues. As I mused about needing to let go of super-ficiality to grasp the deeper meaning and beauty in life, . . . I was vaguely aware that my lips felt numb.

Ignoring the numbness and writing it off to a tight-fitting mask, I continued my snorkeling reverie until I swam over a jellyfish and got stung. This sent me back to the mother ship for some first aid. Once aboard the ship, I decided to monitor my blood glucose. It was 40. My numb lips should have warned me about a low blood sugar.

How humbling.

Lesson number two: Don't get so absorbed in the meaning and beauty of a coral reef that you miss the obvious signs of hypoglycemia.

Amen.

Habits can be good and bad. Habits can be very helpful, for example, blood glucose monitoring that becomes as much a daily habit as toothbrushing. Habits can be destructive when they involve smoking, drinking, or eating to manage stress. Make a list of some of the habits you are aware of in your life. Then, consider the following thoughts about habits to assist you in abolishing bad habits and creating helpful ones.

Habits are at first cobwebs, then, cables.
—Spanish proverb

Habit is a cable; we weave a thread of it every day, and at last we cannot break it.
—Horace Mann

A man is a slave to whatever has mastered him.
—II Peter 2:19

We are what we repeatedly do. Excellence, then, is not an act, but a habit.
—Aristotle

We first make our habits, and then our habits make us.
—John Dryden

Read meditatively. What are the threads you weave daily? Are you a slave to any activity or routine? What is it that you repeatedly do? What healthy habits could you repeatedly do? Then, what would they make you?

As you move through diabetes barriers and challenges toward the goals you hold in your heart, keep in mind:

FAITH   HOPE   CLARITY

Have faith.

Hold tightly to your faith. Know the source of your faith and reconnect with your spiritual roots regularly.

Have hope.

Revisit the cherished stories that keep the flame of hope burning.

Hope, like the gleaming tapers light,
Adorns and cheers our way;
And still, as darker grows the night,
Emits a brighter ray.

–Oliver Goldsmith

Have clarity.

Be clear about who you are, what you want, and where you are going. Good advice from your health care team is your map. A blood glucose meter is your compass. It is you who decide on your destination. With faith, hope, and clarity, you are more likely to get there and reap the rewards of a full life.

Just as our ancestors had to tend to the fire to keep their families warm, fed, and protected, so must we tend to our individual, inner fire. Managing diabetes day after day gets wearying and, sometimes, discouraging, when our results are different from what we had hoped. It is our inner "fire" that creates and sustains enthusiasm (literally defined as God within), energy, faith, hope, and joy.

Fuel for that inner fire comes in many forms. Consider the following, then make your own list.

- worship services
- music and other arts
- friends and the experience of friendship
- service to others
- prayer
- giving our unique gifts to help others
- meaningful work
  (including volunteer work)
- vacations
- inspiring reading with time to reflect
  and process

What have you done recently that fanned the flames of your inner fire? What do you have planned for the near future? Which activities are ongoing?

Don't let this be left up to chance. Tend to your fire.

In the December 1997 *Diabetes Forecast* magazine of the American Diabetes Association, Dr. Robert Tattersall of England made this insightful observation: "Technology has greatly improved the lives of people with diabetes, but it is clearly not a cure-all." Quoting Nobel Prize winner George Minot, Tattersall agreed that what is needed is to "teach the art of courageous living."

Great art conceals great art. The breathtaking beauty of ballet conceals the sweat and aching muscles that went into making the dance look effortless. Whether the artist is dancing, painting, playing music, or throwing pots, there is "art" hidden in the creation of the visible product. This hidden art is the artist's energy, devotion, and skill.

Courageous living is an art, not a science. There are no formulas or recipes. We create by doing. We create a courageous life by trusting, believing, and working hard with the gift of life that we have been given. Most likely, the only visible sign is the life itself. But in moments of quiet reflection, we are aware of the invisible beauty in it—the spiritual dimension—and the Artist's genius.

We are the clay, and thou art our potter; we are all the work of thy hand.

–Isaiah 64:8

Cars, appliances, watches, radios—lots of things come to us with guarantees. We easily and understandably develop an expectation for guarantees in all of life . . . even for Life itself.

Life comes with no guarantees.

We learned that when the diagnosis of diabetes was made. But that didn't end our expectation of some guarantee. When we know people who have lived 50 and 60 years with diabetes, we claim that expectation of longevity. Then we hear of someone who had a heart attack before age 30 or 40 or 50.

And, we learn, again, that we have no guarantees about life.

The blessing in what could be a frightening and frustrating situation is the recognition that life, each day, each moment, is precious. Thus blessed, we stop living in the tomorrow that no one is promised. We live today.

And, if we are truly wise, we LIVE today . . . each day.

In the opening ceremony of the 1988 International Diabetes Federation meeting in Sydney, Australia, a doctor quoted from Shakespeare's *Julius Caesar*. He said:

> *The fault, dear Brutus, lies not in the stars, but in ourselves . . . .*

Read meditatively and apply this thought to your life. Do you see where the opposite could also be true? Our "answers" lie not outside of us, but within us? Do you have personal qualities that make diabetes management difficult? What are the personal qualities that help you meet the challenges of managing diabetes?

Faults may lie within us but so do answers.

In his poem *Psalm of Life*, Henry Wadsworth Longfellow reminds us that we leave behind us "footprints on the sand of time." Further, he suggests that our footprints can be the encouragement for a lost traveler to keep going.

Have you ever felt that you are alone with the challenges you face? Do you know how good it feels to find people who have truly walked in the same moccasins? But, if you find yourself alone, with no one around who has made the journey before you, then, take heart in knowing that it is your footprints that will guide and inspire those who come after you.

Thank you for footprints that have guided my life. Help me to leave footprints that will guide those who follow.

A scholar who had studied Nobel Prize winners shared a remarkable story. He said that all Nobel Prize winners share one unanimously common characteristic: they had all reached a point in their work where they believed they had to give up. Obviously, they shared one more characteristic: they did not give up. Their Nobel Prizes are testimony to the fact that they continued to work.

Winston Churchill adds another dimension to this characteristic by applying it to living with a chronic disease. Most of his life, Churchill struggled with manic depression. This insight into his life makes his famous speech to a group of school children even more inspiring. His ten-word speech was:

Never give up. Never give up. Never, never, never, never.

Experience is not what happens to you; it is what you do with what happens to you.

–Aldous Huxley

In one of his most famous poems, Robert Frost speaks of how taking the road less traveled had made all the difference. I have always believed that Frost was writing about the choices we make and how our choices determine not only the direction but also the quality of our lives.

The experience each of us has with diabetes is largely of our choosing. Each day, each hour of each day, we choose our thoughts and, therefore, our attitudes. We choose our behaviors and experience their consequences. Diabetes "happened." What will you do with it?

At dinner one evening years ago, my husband told me about a new retirement plan for us. Suddenly, I heard myself say, "What? So you can spend it with some cute little blond?" We were both stunned by my uncharacteristic outburst. We finished dinner in a reflective silence.

Days passed, and I took the opportunity to reflect on that scene. I thought about what had happened recently in my life. A diabetic friend of mine had just died at the age of 34 from complications of diabetes. She had graduated Phi Beta Kappa in pharmacy. She had two goals in life: to get married and to get a job. She died without realizing either goal.

Once again I had to come to grips with the loss of a young friend and the reality of my own mortality. At the same time, there was the realization that I am very healthy and have a good chance of living well into retirement. And, the experience connected me once again to my faith. I can only do so much, then I must let go and have faith.

Having come to this awareness, realization, and resolution, I shared it with my husband. Then I said to him, "I don't know about the cute or the little . . . but I have figured out how to stay blond."

Theatre is not about theatre; it is about life.
                                          –Bertolt Brecht

The same can be said of diabetes (or any other chronic disease). For those of us who have it, our interest centers around the meaning diabetes has for daily living and overall satisfaction with life. What impact will diabetes have on my daily life? How will diabetes affect my ability to engage fully in an active and fulfilling life?

Sometimes health care professionals get caught up in the medical meaning of diabetes. Their response to the question: "What does diabetes mean?" may center on glucose metabolism.

I am grateful for my mother's answer that diabetes meant I would live a healthier, more disciplined life. When I asked her what diabetes meant, I was not looking for a scientific or medical response. I wanted her to tell me about me. She helped me to believe that I could always participate fully in life.

Diabetes is not about diabetes; it is about life.

God gave us memories so that we might have roses in December.

—Sir James Barrie

I have enjoyed learning from the people who attend my seminars how it is that they keep their roses well into December. One woman said that she finds it a real boost to keep photographs from vacations in a photo album so that she can revisit the places, cherish the memories. Another person described how enjoyable and uplifting a weekly coffee club has become. He said that members of the group share stories of their families, their vacations, their experiences . . . to be enjoyed again and again. The story was fresh in June, fun to remember in December!

In our school district, there is a program that brings together senior citizens and school children. The seniors' stories provide beautiful roses, the fragrance of which is enjoyed by both groups.

When my nephew Scott died, his wife, Sheila, was 30 years old, and their daughter, Maggie, was six months old. Sheila's friends said to her, "What a pity that Maggie will never know her daddy." Others said, "In the long run, it will be better for Maggie that she simply never even knew Scott."

Sheila's remarkable response to her friends was, "Look, it doesn't matter whether it's 'good' or 'bad.' It's the way it is."

As is true of most profound thoughts, I found other ways to apply this universal truth. Years ago when I spoke to audiences of people who have diabetes, I spoke to them as if I were a cheerleader selling them on the healthy lifestyle that diabetes requires. But it really doesn't matter whether people find the lifestyle requirements to be good or bad. *It's the way it is*. The task for each person is to figure out how to deal constructively with the reality of diabetes.

A diabetes educator in Hawaii told me that the first thing that happens in appointments with patients who have diabetes is that they "talk story." This is the ancient and important practice of conversation, of sharing-the-self, of connecting.

How insightful of Hawaiian practitioners to realize that they are dealing with whole people and cannot focus only on the physical aspects of diabetes. Blood vessels, organs, and nerves do not get diabetes. People do. Whole, intricate, complex human beings. In the process of telling our stories, we gain insights into who we are, and we share that insight with the people who can help us to weave diabetes into our lives.

After the educator told me about this practice, I commented that it might be Hawaiian, but it sounded broader than that. It sounds human. As a storyteller, an experience I always have when I tell stories is that people want to tell theirs.

We are all storytellers. Other's stories are how we learn of the universality of the human experience. We realize that we can and should "talk story" not only in Hawaii but also in Vermont and Mississippi and Arizona and Oregon.

Using urine testing results to manage diabetes is like driving a car by looking in the rearview mirror. All you know is where you've been.
                                    –Dr. Sanford Smith

Dr. Smith's remark made me laugh with delight at a creative, wise description of the old way of testing glucose in urine. As I considered this comment further, I felt thankful for the progress I have experienced in the more than 40 years that I have had diabetes. Because of blood glucose monitoring, I can know where I am and can make wise decisions for moving forward in a positive direction . . . safely and comfortably. Actually, I prefer driving a car by looking forward through the windshield.

Knowledge is not power, it is only potential power that becomes real through use.

–Dorothy Riley

Consider the following statement:

"I know how to monitor my blood glucose. I know how to adjust my food and exercise to keep blood glucose balanced. I know when I can handle diabetes management, and I know when I need to call my health care team for help. I know a lot about diabetes and its management. But, if I do not act on that knowledge, I am no better off than the person who knows nothing."

Would you describe this statement as true or false? Why? How do these thoughts apply to you?

To ask well is to know much.

–African proverb

To gain knowledge we must ask questions. Because we live better with diabetes when we know how to manage it, we need to consider how to ask questions well. That's why many of us write down our questions before each health care appointment. Some clinics even have forms they give out to patients to help them identify the questions they need answered.

Consider your questions. Do they get to the heart of the real issues? Is your question about the amount of fat in your meal plan reflecting a deeper concern about the amount of fat in your blood . . . and your family's history of heart disease? Perhaps "asking well" includes asking more completely. Complete questions include those issues that have to do with the physical concerns (Which protein source is lowest in fat?) as well as mental and spiritual concerns (How can I avoid being so worried about my heart?).

Ask well. Know much. Live better.

Who you are is where you were when.

That is the title of a training film used in the business world. It speaks to how we are shaped by our culture. Those of us who grew up during the 1950s were constantly reminded to eat all of our food because there were starving children in China. Being a member of the "clean plate club" was a great virtue.

Then, diabetes became part of who we are.

Living well with diabetes requires that our various cultural influences are carefully considered in terms of their impact on our diabetes management. Is it useful to belong to the clean plate club? (Was it ever?) What are today's cultural influences on your eating?

When my son was in first grade, he was taught about the different food groups and how important it is to include all of them in a well-balanced meal plan. He came to the dinner table one night and said: "OK, so where are all the food groups?"

What are the cultural messages in your life today? How do they influence you?

Sailing is a bit of a mystery to me. I am fascinated to watch sailboats crisscross, back and forth across the water, sometimes with the wind and sometimes against it. When I heard a description of what sailors do, I saw that their approach to sailing is very similar to a successful approach to diabetes management.

Sailors do not fight the wind, neither do they ignore it and hope that it will simply blow itself into the sail and move the boat. They understand the wind, and they have skills in sailing. They use their knowledge and experience to their advantage. They catch the wind through skilled techniques and make it work for them.

What do we do with blood glucose? Like wind providing the fuel for a sailboat, blood glucose provides the "fuel" for our bodies . . . if we use our knowledge, skill, and experience.

I discovered I always have choices, and sometimes it's only a choice of attitude.

–Abraham Lincoln

The greater danger for most of us is not that our aim is too high and we miss it, but that it is too low and we reach it.

–Michelangelo

An aphorism is a short, concise statement of a principle. Perhaps it is precisely because of their brevity that aphorisms can be remembered and used as a reflective springboard to help people dive into the depth of their own experiences, memories, and stories.

Where do these two aphorisms take you?

What are your favorite quotes?

Dr. Viktor Frankl wrote *Man's Search for Meaning* drawing on his experiences as a psychiatrist and a survivor of Nazi concentration camps. Frankl believed that "decisions, not conditions" are what mental health is about. He also felt strongly that people do not get better by seeing themselves as a victim.

Some questions to consider: If diabetes is the "condition," then what are the decisions that we can make to achieve mental health? The second question is: Do you see yourself as a victim or a victor?

Listen to your self-talk. What are the messages that you give yourself? Would you characterize them as being more life-affirming? Or self-defeating?

Finally, what decision can you make that will help you to see yourself as a victor?

A bad messenger plunges men into trouble, but a faithful envoy brings healing.

–Proverbs 13:17

A diabetes educator recalled meeting with a man newly diagnosed with diabetes. The man told the educator that he knew all about diabetes, about the complications he would experience, about his early death. His wife cried.

The startled educator asked him where he had learned about diabetes. He showed her a book that had been written 30 years earlier. The educator immediately began an up-to-date education that was, of course, far more hopeful.

Education is a never-ending process. We need to make sure that we have good resources for our education.

A diabetes educator friend of mine told me that keeping a journal is the way that she discovers her spiritual self. She said that the journal is the place we realize how consistently we spin out the same webs only to be re-caught in them.

What an interesting thought! Is the spinning of a web similar to the setting of a goal? Have you ever set a goal (weight loss, regular exercise, meditative reading) only to find yourself re-setting that goal some weeks or months later? That's what getting "re-caught" in the same webs means to me.

Identify a goal that you set for yourself in the past year. If you did not reach the goal, explore why. Why do you find yourself re-caught in the same web? What will you do differently this time so you can achieve the goal?

My friend learned a big lesson when the family cat had kittens. He learned that life isn't fair. It can be very painful. (The kittens were immediately given away.) And he learned that food is very comforting. Bob's mother gave all the children chocolate sundaes the day the kittens left home.

As an adult, Bob found himself very overweight. He observed his behavior. He realized that whenever he felt stressed, he ate. Food not only comforts, too much of it makes you fat. So, he chose to make exercise his stress manager.

Around the time that I heard this story about Bob, my 4-year-old son, John, and I were shopping and became separated. When we finally found each other, we had a tearful reunion. Then, I took him to the bakery and bought him a cookie. As he was putting the cookie up to his sweet little mouth, I thought about my friend's experience and realized, with horror, that I was teaching my son that "cookies make owies go away." From that point on, I intentionally avoided food as a comfort and a reward for my son.

When the family dog died, I called a former neighbor and we told "Max" stories, laughing at the memories, crying over his loss . . . all the while healing. I told my son how I had handled the pain I experienced. I did not offer him food. I hugged him and told him about what had helped me. There are healthy, helpful ways to manage stress.

Max fathered ten puppies before he died. John knows where all of them are. Max's grandson could be in our future.

My Canadian grandmother read tea leaves. Nana could predict when she would get company and what the weather was likely to be.

I practice a more common reverie; I read clouds. The reading of clouds is not for predictions of future events. Reading clouds can be an enjoyable way to pass an hour or two on a summer afternoon or a pleasant, relaxing way to engage in the important act of self-reflection. And, because we gaze heavenward when we watch clouds, this could also be an opportunity for meditation—that is, listening to what God is saying to us.

Take time. Quiet yourself. Listen.

Robert Louis Stevenson is said to have had tuberculosis most of his life. His philosophy for living with a chronic disease can be seen in his statement:

Life is not a matter of holding good cards. It's playing a poor hand well.

Each of us decides how to play our cards. The experience of having diabetes is largely of our own choosing.

The experience can be one of deprivation and difficulty.

The experience of living with diabetes can be one of growth and healthful living.

We choose our actions and our attitudes. What are your actions and attitudes when you are playing the hand of diabetes well?

I need wisdom, grace, and courage to play my hand well.

We don't receive wisdom; we must discover it for ourselves after a journey that no one can take for us or spare us.

—Marcel Proust

The Search Institute in Minneapolis has done research into the personal assets that young people need to avoid high-risk behaviors.

Our search is for the personal assets we need to live well with the challenge of diabetes. Research and personal experience have led me to believe that these assets include:

A positive attitude
The ability to solve problems
A positive self-image
Faith in a higher power
Effective stress management
The capacity to adapt
Self-discipline
Motivation
Hope

What are the assets that have helped you? How did you discover them?

In the Fall as we harvest wisdom, let's look at the process of learning. A scientist looks at every experiment as a lesson from which to learn. When an experiment doesn't work, the scientist may say, "I tried. It didn't work, but I learned something." This leads to a philosophy that there is no failure, only lessons.

When I received my first blood glucose meter, I experimented by having an ice cream cone . . . dipped in chocolate. The resulting blood glucose was well over 200. I learned. Each day I am my own personal scientist . . . learning, one experiment at a time.

Wisdom comes to us lesson by lesson.

*Quiet minds cannot be perplexed or frightened
but go on in fortune or misfortune at their own
private pace like the ticking of a clock during a
thunderstorm.*

−Robert Louis Stevenson

Our busy lives, numerous daily stresses, and concerns often produce a mental state in us that is anything but quiet. Yet, most of us acknowledge that peace of mind is highly desirable.

Once in a great while, we experience peace that just settles over us like the afghan that Grandma used to throw over us when we were napping on the sofa. More often, if we are to experience peace of mind, we must seek it.

The Psalms are full of peace. Consider focusing on this thought:

*Wait for the Lord; be strong, and let your heart
take courage.*

−Psalm 27:14

Wait for the Lord; be strong, and let your heart take
Wait for the Lord; be strong, and let your heart
Wait for the Lord; be strong, and let your
Wait for the Lord; be strong, and let
Wait for the Lord; be strong, and
Wait for the Lord; be strong,
Wait for the Lord; be
Wait for the Lord;
Wait for the
Wait for
Wait

Sometimes people say they are really counting on a cure for diabetes in their lifetime. Most of us hope for one. All of us would probably welcome it. But, counting on a cure can be dangerous if it means that diabetes is not well-managed because a person is relying on a cure to escape long-term complications.

My position during 40 years of diabetes has been to manage diabetes to the best of my ability so that when a cure does become available, I will be in the best possible health.

A statement in the book *Active Spirituality* by Charles R. Swindoll offers insight into what happens when people pray for a cure. "When we fully rely upon the Lord to handle a given situation, He may, in his ultimate wisdom, remove all the obstacles and smooth out our path thoroughly. Or He may choose, instead, to walk with us along the rocky path."

There is comfort in that. Even if a cure is not found in our lifetime, we will not walk the rocky path of diabetes alone.

Life's mysteries may defy our understanding, but still we seek meaning. That's where philosophy, faith, and the arts come into play in our lives. We may never understand why we got diabetes, but we can find meaning in our experience with it.

Practical lessons that diabetes can teach us include the importance of goal setting, problem solving, and stress management. Spiritual meaning can come from numerous sources. Corrie ten Boom, author and survivor of the Holocaust, explained how she thinks about problems in life that defy understanding.

Picture a piece of embroidery placed between you and God, with the right side up toward God.
Man sees the loose, frayed ends; but God sees the pattern.

How can a thread like diabetes add to the beauty of Life's tapestry?

The daughter of a friend of mine has a handicapped child. When he was born, his handicap was a total surprise and a great shock. I wrote her a letter and shared all that I have to share, my heart. In part, the letter said:

"I believe that pain is never totally erased. We keep transcending it by God's grace and love. This love is expressed through family, friends, other families who share the same or similar challenge . . . and at some truly remarkable point, we begin to receive His power and love by *giving* it ourselves. That is the greatest blessing and, I believe, the sign that healing is really occurring. You can't rush the process. Perhaps the point I most want to share with you is TRUST that you will get to that healing that allows you to transcend pain. God bless you with strength, love, laughter, tears, comfort, wisdom, power, and joy as you travel on your journey."

Shared sorrow is sorrow cut in half; shared joy is doubled.

—Swedish proverb

Our efforts to "get over" the tragic or unpleasant events of life are misspent. People don't ever get over the major traumas of their lives. These events shape us and the way we view life. Once we have experienced tragedy, it becomes a thread in the fabric of our life. However, we can choose whether that thread strengthens or weakens our fabric.

Our task is to find the meaning these experiences hold for us and use their lessons to heal ourselves and others. In observing people who have experienced tragedy, I have seen one common characteristic in the people who appear to make the most progress in healing. They focus on love instead of loss. Their "fabric" becomes stronger as their love strengthens others.

Dave spends a day a week volunteering at the hospital where his son, Scott, died.

Jean, whose daughter Julie died, writes a book with her pastor on spiritual issues in adolescents' lives.

Linda and Rich, who lost their daughter, Laura, build a healing garden . . . for the whole community.

Reflect on your response to tragedy you have known. It's not too late to move toward love.

The pace of life seems to be a major source of stress for many of us. Even people who have retired talk about being too busy . . . too much to do . . . never enough time. The late Norman Vincent Peale wrote a lovely essay on "Taking Time to Live." In it he said:

Do not be a slave to life's machinery; get a beautiful song, a lovely poem, and the whisper of God into your soul.

Do you know where your resources are that give you spiritual nourishment? Look in the basement, the attic, or on your bookshelves. Many of us have books that we've had for many years and haven't read in some time. I am so grateful that I hung on to all my textbooks in American, English, and world literature. Even the things I've read before offer new insights—an unexpected beauty.

Marcel Proust must have had in mind all these wonderful thinkers and writers when he wrote:

Let us be grateful to people who make us happy; they are the charming gardeners who make our souls blossom.

The title of an article in the *Harvard Business Review* gave me an insight into diabetes management. The title was: "Management by Whose Objectives?" The business community has long realized that the corporate goal will be achieved if individuals are allowed to set and achieve *their own* goals.

The way I see the corporate goal for diabetes is the overall goal of well-managed diabetes. For that goal to be achieved, the individuals who have diabetes must be able to pursue their personal goals. Sometimes it may seem that health care professionals have blood glucose management as their only goal . . . while we who have diabetes are interested in the day-to-day enjoyment of life.

Ultimately, we do have the same goal. That is why we need to communicate our values, needs, and other goals to our health care providers. Diabetes management is a team effort. Diabetes will get managed based on the objectives held by the person who has diabetes and with the counsel and advice of the health care team.

I like my diabetes team. They consider me the central member of the team. They are there to help me achieve the objectives I have for my life.

Having a supportive health care team is absolutely essential to living well with the challenge of diabetes. Because diabetes needs to be managed on a daily, and even hourly, basis, we need support available to us outside of the clinic . . . in the laboratory of life. I am inspired by the stories of people around me who are generous enough to share how they support one another.

A retired teacher friend of ours is just such a generous and loving person. He told of the experience that he and his wife had when she was being treated for cancer, and gave us insight into the remarkable human capacity to cope. Commenting on her baldness following chemotherapy, he said, "There's more of her to kiss."

My friend and mentor, Reverend Robert Esbjornson, is well-acquainted with diabetes. His daughter has had it for more than 40 years, his son has had it for 20 years, and his wife had it for many years prior to her death from breast cancer.

His perspective includes not only that of a person standing by, but also a professional with more than 30 years experience as a professor of medical ethics. He has thought deeply about life with diabetes. One conclusion he has reached is that the basic strategy for care is not that of a warrior making war on an ailment. Rather, we are the diplomat engaged in ongoing negotiations, accepting the condition as a fact that won't go away but that can be managed.

Diplomacy, not war. Negotiating with finesse, not fighting.

What role do you play in managing diabetes? Warrior? Diplomat? Other?

Birth and death are present in every moment.
                                    –Thich Nhat Hanh

At the end of the play *Cyrano de Bergerac*, an old, frail Cyrano is seated beneath a tree while leaves gracefully fall down around him. The falling leaves give beauty, gentleness, and a naturalness to Cyrano's impending death. Leaves let go and fall without regret. This seasonal metaphor helps us to realize that death is not final. New life emerges from the old in another season.

Plays, poetry, music . . . the arts . . . are gifts of the spirit. Their messages lodge in our hearts and surface at times later in life when we need their instruction, insight, inspiration, and healing.

Meditations on Diabetes

*Every moment Nature starts on the longest
journey, and every moment she reaches her goal.*
                                        –Goethe

Each day we race toward Life's "finish line." It is well to pause and make note of where we are. Although you may not see this point in your journey as your version of the finish line, where you are is its own endpoint. It is a place of beauty, a place with lessons to share, joy to give, and growth to experience.

Traditional Chinese medicine promotes living in the moment, being "present" in the moment. This philosophy is greatly enhanced by the fact that the Chinese language has no past or future tense. Everything is present.

Carry that thought with you today. Each moment is its own destination.

The battles that count aren't the ones for gold medals. The struggles within yourself—the invisible, inevitable battles inside all of us—that's where it's at.

—Jesse Owens

Diabetes is largely an invisible disease. People cannot tell by looking at us that we have diabetes. The term *invisible chronicity* applies to diabetes and any other chronic condition that cannot be seen. Because our diabetes is not apparent to the people around us, the challenges we encounter in managing it are taken on within ourselves.

I have always felt a tremendous admiration for people who have diabetes. Few people understand what it means, what we do, what we face.

I think we all deserve gold medals.

Let everyone sweep in front of her own door and the whole world will be clean.

—Goethe

At times, the health care picture in this country is painted as so grim and hopeless that we individuals are left feeling helpless to effect any positive change. But, as individuals, we can positively impact our own health, that of our families, and, ultimately, that of our country. Our day-to-day choices make a difference in our own lives, and when we multiply healthy choices by many individuals, the impact is great.

A woman aboard an airplane had a seizure because of low blood sugar. She was taken off the plane by paramedics, taken by ambulance to a hospital, and kept overnight. She had taken her insulin that morning but didn't eat enough food. A totally preventable problem had cost the "system" thousands of dollars.

A man in a restaurant took his insulin after being told that his wait would be about 30 minutes. An hour and a half later, he awakened with a paramedic bending over him.

Today, diabetes is one of the most expensive diseases in our nation. One in seven health care dollars is spent on diabetes. Before Medicare limits how many blood glucose strips they will allow people to have, let's look at other ways to cut costs.

Preventable problems are just that—preventable. Let each of us commit to taking charge of our lives, taking responsibility for our choices. Our choices can save the system money; our choices can enhance our health and future well-being.

Winter

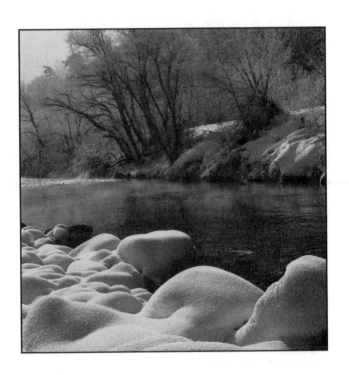

Introduction to Winter

Winter can be a cozy time—a time to curl up by the fire and listen to music. Winter is traditionally a reflective sort of season—the days are short, the weather can be cold—a good time to sit by the hearth of your mind and look into the fire of your soul.

> *Who looks outside dreams, who looks inside wakes.*
>
> –Carl Jung

For me, courage is the overall theme of Winter. Outside it is cold and nothing grows. It is dark. There is little out there to sustain us. Winter is the season we experience whenever tragedy hits. We are forced to depend on our inner resources. It takes courage to look inside oneself. To what will you awaken if you "look inside?" By not looking inside, do you run the risk of dreaming your life away? Winter continues the theme of this book of asking questions—not to receive answers but to receive insights. That's how I interpret Jung's statement. We awaken to insights that help to challenge, inspire, and guide us through the tough times.

Meditations on Diabetes

Courage is surely necessary when life confronts us with pain, unpredictable events, isolation— life's proverbial "what ifs"—and the common, painful experience of the loss of a dream. In the Winter meditations, you are invited to explore what courage means to you and how you can tap into the "well of courage" deep within you—as well as receive inspiration from examples of courage around you.

How do you see courage? A roaring lion? A tall, resolute pine tree? A toddler picking herself up after a fall? A person injecting insulin for the first time? For the hundredth or ten thousandth time? "See" the image of courage as you understand it.

Hear the voices of courage: Martin Luther King, Jr., the prophet Isaiah, Louisa May Alcott, Lucille Ball, Eleanor Roosevelt, a soldier in the Persian Gulf, Robert Fulghum, Henry Wadsworth Longfellow, Reinhold Niebuhr, Rabbi Abraham Heschel, and Joseph Campbell.

Understand your life in the context of the lives of other courageous people. You are courage.

In the midst of lonely days and dreary nights I have heard an inner voice saying, "Lo, I will be with you."

–Martin Luther King, Jr.

For centuries, the "inner voice" has been written about and revered for the guidance and the mysterious, peaceful assurance it gives believers. We have all known lonely days and dreary nights, though probably few of us have experienced dreary nights with the profound pain that Dr. King did. Still, we each learn our own lessons.

The words from Dr. King's quote that jump out at me are, "I have heard." He didn't say, "I have read about" or "I have been told about." He said, "I have heard an inner voice."

That inner voice is within you, within me, within all of us. Let us focus in this Winter section on listening for the still, small voice within.

Pause again today.   Listen.

Meditation is a form of reflection with a spiritual focus. While prayer can be defined as talking to God, meditation is listening to God. Connecting with the spirit and the spiritual requires meditation. Robert Esbjornson, retired religion professor, talks of a "meditative style" as a way of paying attention while you are reading, writing, conversing—even eating and exercising—that opens people to the more or less obscure world of the soul.

Meditative listening is similar to reading to find deeper meaning and opens us to messages we may miss in conversation. So often we hear or see the words but not the wisdom. Bob's advice is: "Listen for something that touches your soul."

The next step is to engage in meditative writing. People write as a response to what they are reading or hearing. The writing can be directed to yourself, the author, or God. Meditative writing can help to clarify your thoughts and beliefs. All of these meditative activities are part of what Esbjornson refers to as "meditative intention," which keeps you aware so your reading and conversing bear spiritual fruit.

Listen . . . .

As a father and a husband, Bob Esbjornson has described himself as "standing by" family members who have chronic diseases. With eloquence and heart-felt understanding, he describes *his* needs.

He says, "I need up-to-date information about these illnesses, what the illnesses are, what treatments are available, what prognosis of future developments are realistic. Information is not enough for me, however. I also need the nurture of my moral disposition, because dealing with chronic illnesses can be discouraging and frustrating. Moral qualities are inner conditions, to be sure, but they are exhaustible and need nourishment from beyond the self.

"This nourishment comes from the support of wise and understanding and compassionate people among one's family and friends; and from ethical and religious teachings that can be practiced until they become habits of the heart."

For the many millions of people who have diabetes, there are many more millions of people who are directly affected because they are family members or friends. All people who are affected by diabetes need nourishment for their hearts and souls. If you are a person standing by family members who have diabetes, how well are you being nourished? If you are the person with diabetes, what evidence do you see that the people standing by you are getting the nourishment they need?

There are two ways to live your life. One is as though nothing is a miracle. The other is as though everything is a miracle.

–Albert Einstein

Quite naturally people have favorite seasons: winter for skiers, spring for gardeners, summer for boaters, and fall for hikers. The favorite seasons in our lives might be defined by ages or events. Some we like better than others. But the truly wise person has discovered what Albert Einstein did: everything is a miracle.

Only when life is approached with this perspective, do the miracles reveal themselves. The person who grumbles about having to watch a toddler misses the wonder and delight in her discoveries.

Those of us who live with a health challenge may think of the pre-illness days as the preferred season in life, but we do so at the risk of closing ourselves off from the day-to-day miracles happening now. I cannot choose to live my life without diabetes. I can choose to see the miracle in blood glucose monitoring, an insulin infusion pump, and the effects of exercise on my body.

**Help me to be open
to the miracles that surround me.**

For many years, the darkest, most difficult day of my life with diabetes was the day of my annual dilated eye exam. I dreaded going, yet remained faithful to making the appointment, year after year.

I had difficulty because I was afraid that the ophthalmologist would discover eye disease. I didn't want to go blind. Ironically, I thought of not making an appointment . . . but, logic always prevailed. To ignore eye exams meant putting my head in the sand. Denial can be dangerous. Denial of problems does not make them go away. Worse yet, denial could lead to missing the early treatment that could save my eyesight.

As I grew in spirit over the years, fear dissolved into a healthy concern that, miraculously, evolved into peace. The wisdom of the prophet Isaiah helped to direct my focus for each eye appointment.

Thou dost keep him in perfect peace, whose mind is stayed on thee, because he trusts in thee.
            –Isaiah 26:3

After 27 years of imprisonment, Nelson Mandela was asked how it felt to be free. His response was: "I have always been free."

Some people see diabetes as a power struggle. They see their struggle for control as a tug-of-war between them and the disease.

At the diagnosis of diabetes when I was ten years old, I drew the proverbial line in the sand, and let it be known that I would be in control. Hospitalized nearly two weeks, I had to endure painful attempts to find blood in the hidden veins of my right arm. (My left arm was covered with a plaster cast.) Although I could not control the daily blood-letting, I made an important decision. With tears streaming into my ears as I lay in the hospital bed, I decided that I would get married in a state that did not require a blood test. There would be one blood test I could control. I felt empowered. I felt free.

And, even though there have been many blood tests over the years, I have never lost the feeling that I am in control. At a very young age, I had learned that the most important control I could have was control over my thoughts.

**Help me to make life-affirming choices . . .
beginning with my thoughts.**

A spiritual winter can blow into town in any month. The tell-tale signs of "frost" include despairing statements like these:

"I am working out regularly, and I still don't have the toned body I want."

"I'm monitoring blood glucose levels, making the best decisions I can, and I still have highs and lows."

Without predictable outcomes, how does one keep going? Day after day after day?

Faithfulness
Living *by* values, not *for* results.

Is it possible that:
Faith is more important than outcomes?
Frustration can teach me patience?
My steadfast determination will inspire others?
Disappointment actually strengthens me?
Success, when it comes, will be even sweeter because of my struggles?
"Success" may have an entirely new and deeper meaning?

It is possible.
So, I keep going.

I am not afraid of storms, for I am learning how to sail my ship.

—Louisa May Alcott

One of the gifts we can receive from diabetes is self-confidence. Unless or until we experience difficulty in life, we really don't know how we will respond. When we learn how to navigate through the "storm" of diabetes, we gain a self-confidence that helps us with any of life's challenges.

Like sailing, diabetes requires specific skills. Nutrition education helps us to navigate through grocery stores and restaurants. Exercise education leads us to explore what type, how much, how often, and the very important question: what do I enjoy? The "meds" in diabetes education include "medication" to address physical need and "meditation" to meet mental and spiritual needs.

To sail the ship of diabetes successfully we need to know the physical information. Equally important is psychological, social, and spiritual hardiness to take on any of the storms that life presents.

When we discover that we can manage diabetes, then we gain a boost of self-confidence. The blessing in this self-confidence is that it does carry over to other life challenges. We've handled one; we can handle another.

Give me courage to navigate through all of life's storms . . . especially the ones I may face today.

Meditations on Diabetes

A woman stranded alone at night on a mountain in freezing temperatures and falling snow on Christmas Eve knew it was dance or die. So, she danced in the dark, playing tunes in her head, until dawn Christmas Day, when rescuers found her.

She danced to keep warm, to stay awake . . . to live.

What a wonderfully heroic story! As I read it in the newspaper, I thought of the times over the years when I have been stranded in various places . . . usually airports. I thought about how grateful I was to have my blood glucose meter, insulin, and extra food. I've always made it through these experiences . . . sometimes with a begrudging spirit. This story helped me to see that I can do more than merely "make it." I can survive with joy . . . with body, mind, and soul intact.

Along with granola bars, I shall add music to my survival kit.

Nothing endures but personal qualities.

–Walt Whitman

In his poem *What Endures*, Walt Whitman reminded me that nothing outside of me is as great as the qualities that lie within me. This process of self-reflection is at the heart of the power of poetry and is, I believe, its purpose.

The libraries in our communities hold many books of poetry. Now, when poetry is no longer our school assignment, perhaps we can return to poetry on purpose and discover . . . ourselves.

Bring me to the words that will nourish my mind and spirit.

In reading this meditatively, consider the following questions:

- What are personal qualities? honesty? steadfastness? kindness?
- What are my personal qualities?
- How is it that personal qualities endure?
- Why is that important?

Winter is a metaphor. It can represent difficulties, loneliness, darkness, cold, and despair. We all are vulnerable to a winter spirit. Spiritual winters can hit us any time, even on a bright, sunny day in July.

However, when a dreary spirit comes on us on a cold, blustery, cloudy day in January, we feel that blast of winter doubly hard. Mental health experts talk about seasonal affective disorder (SAD) causing depression in the winter because of the short days and the lack of sunlight. An antidote is to increase the light in one's surroundings. I have at least one extra lamp turned on in our living room all winter. Perhaps that helps prevent the physical disorder.

My spiritual light comes from music, laughter, poetry, and prayer.

**Beam your light into the dark corners
of my heart. Thank you.**

If you are patient in one moment of anger, you will escape a hundred days of sorrow.

–Chinese proverb

The diagnosis of diabetes can be viewed as the loss of a dream. Most of us have dreams about what we want our lives to be. Few people would include a chronic disease like diabetes. The work of Elisabeth Kübler-Ross identified a process that people experience when they lose a loved one. The process is similar when you lose a dream—disbelief, anger, sadness, denial, alternating hopefulness and hopelessness, and finally, acceptance.

Psychologists can help people who get "stuck" in the process, finding it difficult to take the steps from anger to acceptance. Many people find their own path to healing. The mother of a young girl with diabetes told me that once in awhile, her daughter gets fed up with having to have injections of insulin. Her path to healing began with making a small pile of used, plastic, disposable syringes with the needles clipped. She would proceed to stamp her feet again and again on the syringes, venting her anger, and shedding her tears until she felt better.

What rituals do you use to vent your anger? Hitting a golf ball? Punching a pillow? Engaging in strenuous physical activity? Writing out your thoughts, and then, ceremoniously tearing up the paper?

Anger is a natural feeling. It is neither good nor bad; it just is. How we handle anger is what makes this emotion a destructive force or an empowering one. Reflect on recent experiences with anger. How did these experiences make you feel? What did you choose to do?

The last of the human freedoms—to choose one's attitude in any given set of circumstances—is to choose one's own way.

—Victor Frankl

Following a presentation that I had just given to a group of people who have diabetes, a delightful, older gentleman approached me. With twinkling eyes and a huge smile, he spoke: "Do you know what my pappy always said?" Of course, I didn't, but I was so excited, because I knew that he was going to tell me!

"My pappy always said, 'Ya gotta have an attitude of gratitude!'" He told me about his father who had been one of the pioneers in insulin therapy, receiving insulin in the 1920s. Now, in the 1980s, this man was alive because of the miracle of insulin and ALIVE because he chose to be. He had chosen an attitude of gratitude.

Each day each of us is faced with choosing what our attitude is going to be. We certainly don't always choose our circumstances. Victor Frankl was in a Nazi concentration camp during World War II. He lost everything. He could make no choices about his life. But, he discovered that he could choose his attitude. He chose to be hopeful. Not only did he survive, he was alive with his sanity and compassion intact.

Philosophers tell us that human growth has its roots in pain. Those who do not experience growth get stuck in a philosophy like this one: "Life's a bitch; then you die." For others, challenges like a chronic disease can become the vehicles to carry them on a journey of self-discovery and growth.

Between these extremes of "Life is difficult" and "Difficulties help me to grow" is a middle ground where the philosophy might be: "This is the way life is, so I'll make the best of it."

The famous figure skater Scott Hamilton had cancer. I saw him skate following his surgery and recovery. He gave a dazzling, energetic, beautiful performance. His inspiring spirit is evident in this statement attributed to him:

The only disability in life is a bad attitude.

I read a newspaper article one winter about the need for winter "comfort foods." Psychologists remind us that eating for comfort can lead to obesity . . . and high blood sugars for people with diabetes. Consider the "comfort foods" that nourish your spirit. One of my favorites is a bouquet of daisies. Fresh flowers in January are so delightfully unexpected that they jolt me into noticing them. Daisies invariably lift my spirits.

Comfort comes from other sources: a talk with a soul mate, a gathering of friends, the familiarity of place (home, club, place of worship), the familiarity of routine (humdrum as "routine" is to us, at times, there is comfort in its steady changelessness). And comfort comes from knowing that the "still small voice" within us will always be there. These are, indeed, nourishment for the spirit—giving us comfort.

What lifts you out of a wintry spirit?

What are your spirit's comfort foods?

A question that is frequently explored by both health care professionals and people who have diabetes is: "What is the primary reason people find it difficult to follow their diabetes regimen?" The question arises from the observation that although people with diabetes know how to manage diabetes, quite often they don't act on that knowledge.

What is your experience with diabetes? When you do find it difficult to follow the regimen of meal plan, regular exercise, medication-taking, and stress management, why is it? What are the barriers?

Some of the insights into this question that I have gathered over the years include barriers, such as a lack of support, a negative set of subcultures, a poor self-image, poor coping mechanisms, feelings of powerlessness, bad habits, hopelessness, and the fact that the disease never goes away, that lead to periodically falling off the wagon, or a reluctance to even get on the wagon.

Awareness of your difficulties is an important step in setting goals. Consider the following affirmation:

I am clear about what my real difficulty is in coping with diabetes.

I have the wisdom to understand the true nature of my challenge.

I have the strength to seek help from health care providers, family, and friends.

I can set goals.

I can solve problems.

As I learn, I grow.

I celebrate life.

Behold I do not give lectures or a little charity.
When I give, I give myself.

–Walt Whitman

Feelings of isolation and loneliness provoke some of our darkest hours. People who don't have diabetes simply do not and cannot understand what it is like to live with diabetes. Even in the midst of loving family and caring friends, we can experience loneliness. We can feel isolated at the clinic even though we are surrounded by caring health care professionals. As helpful and supportive as these important people are, there is still a missing element of personal understanding.

Support groups can fill that need. A support group is a place where wisdom dwells and courage fuels discussion. Generally, humor is ever-present to warm discussion and soften the rough edges of feelings. Confidentiality wraps her arms around the group, and respect presides at every gathering. Sometimes people sit around a table, but they always gather around the campfire of the human heart. Such a support group provides a place where people can tell their stories to listeners who will care, not judge, not offer advice, just listen and care . . . and probably understand.

Consider attending or forming a support group of people interested in living positively with diabetes. Such a group can be organized in neighborhoods, at worksites, and in places of worship. In addition to the spiritual cornerstones of wisdom, courage, humor, and respect, what other qualities do you regard as essential to the building of a support group? In a group, there is both the giving and the receiving of support. Dr. Hans Selye referred to helping others as a very effective way to manage stress. Giving of oneself is the ultimate gift we give to others . . . and ourselves.

One of the things I learned the hard way was it does not pay to get discouraged. Keeping busy and making optimism a way of life can restore your faith in yourself.

–Lucille Ball

Andrea Meade Lawrence was an Olympic alpine skier. In one of her runs down a mountain during Olympic competition, she hit a flag and fell. Without missing a beat, she got up and continued down the mountain. She won the gold medal.

What do you suppose her thoughts were when she hit the flag? "Oh darn. I blew it." That thought could have led her to give up. The fact that she kept going suggests that her thoughts were ones of courage, determination, and faith. She believed she could make it—and she did.

What are your thoughts when you hit a flag in your life, such as experiencing an unexpectedly high or low blood sugar? What helps you keep going? What are the thoughts that help you get up when you're down?

Be strong and of good courage; be not frightened, neither be dismayed; the Lord your God is with you wherever you go.

–Joshua 1:9

Diabetes introduced me to the "what ifs." It's a torturous game that most of us play but few of us win . . . unless you call "winning" the insight that there will always be more questions than answers.

After my son was born, I experienced a new dimension of concerns over what would happen to my family if I were to experience the serious complications of diabetes. I wondered what it would mean to be a blind mother . . . what if . . . what if . . . .

In moments of quiet reflection, I visualized what I could understand of that possibility. At the time of this reflection, my son was a toddler. I was spending a lot of time reading to him. *What if I couldn't read to my child?* The response to that question gave me the peace that I sought. What if my son would read to me, and this experience would strengthen his character?

I could begin to receive peace from these thoughts because I value character development. I continued to receive peace when I thought through the roles that God and I play. I do the best I can to manage my diabetes on a daily basis. He takes all my worries and replaces them with peace . . . if I believe.

I gain strength, courage, and confidence by every experience in which I must stop and look fear in the face.

—Eleanor Roosevelt

Winter can symbolize struggle and difficulties of life . . . like diabetes. The diagnosis experience is often a wintry time in the lives of all the people affected: the person who is diagnosed, family members, and friends. Anger, fear, resentment, and depression are common responses to the diagnosis. And so is courage, the primary spiritual quality of winter.

Courage keeps us going as we travel through our difficulties, exploring our strengths, learning all the lessons that winter has to teach.

What is there to see in the fearful face of diabetes? The complications of blindness, kidney failure, and nerve damage? Strength, courage, and confidence came out of the report of the DCCT, a National Institutes of Health study that showed that a modest improvement in glycohemoglobin results reduced the risk of these complications by half.

We need courage, not to face the complications as if they were inevitable, but courage to live the healthy life that makes them preventable.

As we move through life, there are changing circumstances—from technologies to social trends. This is fertile ground for discovering new lessons about Life.

Computers have introduced quite a few changes to our lives and can help us understand an important lesson about personal choice and responsibility. We have more power when we view ourselves as the programmer, not the program acting out of someone else's design.

We can actually program each day by the goals we set. Sometimes our goals get redirected because Life has other plans for the day. But, at least if we begin each day with goals, we'll start in a direction of our choosing.

Taking responsibility for our choices requires COURAGE. Remind yourself of that when you feel a strong temptation to give in and follow the path of least resistance, someone else's "program." It takes courage to pass up pastries or to take a walk when you don't feel like it.

Think courage; see yourself as courageous; act courageously.

A futurist once made this comment: "No country, corporation, or individual can hope to move forward positively without a positive future self-image." Future is a word that can get clouded over by the uncertainty created by a chronic disease. Courage, certainly, is necessary for anyone living with a chronic disease to be able to believe in a positive future. This belief can also be awakened by stories that show us how we can create the positive future self-image we desire. Consider this story:

> One day a man observed his neighbor in the backyard standing by a huge rock, with hammer and chisel in hand. The man walked over to his neighbor and asked what he was doing. "Oh, I thought I'd try my hand at sculpting," was the reply. The man said to his neighbor, "But you have no training, no experience. You're crazy!" and he left that day on vacation. When he returned two weeks later, he was astounded to see in his neighbor's backyard a perfect sculpture of an elephant. He went directly to his neighbor and demanded, "How'd you do that?!" The humble neighbor shrugged his shoulders and responded, "I don't know, I just chipped away everything that didn't look like an elephant."

Clearly, he needed to know what an elephant looked like to have an accurate visual image of what to sculpt. What is the future self-image you would like? Do you see a healthy, active, well-toned body? Do you see a look on your face that speaks of the peace, joy, and contentment that you feel?

On a day-to-day basis, as you "see" a behavior about to occur that does not lead to the positive future self-image you seek, then chip it away.

We are all sculptors of ourselves.
                                        –Henry David Thoreau

Thoughts create feelings. It is angry thoughts that cause us to feel angry. Peaceful thoughts create a feeling of peace. Consider this concept and check it out for yourself. Whenever you are aware of an identifiable feeling, check on your thoughts. And, if you wish to change a feeling, see what happens when you change your thoughts.

Because words are the basis for thoughts, consider your use of certain words and what thoughts and feelings arise from them. Do you "test" your blood glucose or do you "monitor?" Some of you may say, "It's the same thing." Others will see the difference as significant.

Testing implies pass or fail. The word *test* is judgmental. Since people do not like to fail or feel like a failure, some (out of fear of failure) may not check their blood glucose. However, if you say and think *monitor*, there is quite a different meaning and feeling. To monitor is to seek information. The data collected is used for decision-making, not judging. Your thoughts about blood glucose monitoring can make it a burden or a blessing. Compare these two thoughts:

1) As if age, weight, income, and IQ were not enough, blood glucose results give us another set of numbers by which we can judge ourselves . . . or be judged.

2) Blood glucose monitoring provides me with information that helps me to be in control of my life. I can have greater safety and comfort when I know where my blood glucose level is.

**We can choose our thoughts.
Are yours helpful?**

You cannot prevent the birds of unhappiness from flying overhead, but you can prevent them from building a nest in your hair.

—Chinese proverb

Thoughts can come into our minds, but we do not need to allow them to take up permanent residence! During National Diabetes Month (November), newspapers, radio, and television carry messages that describe the devastating complications of diabetes. Although it is undeniably important for people with diabetes to know about complications and how they are caused, it can be dangerous to focus too much attention on them.

One danger is becoming so fearful of complications that we miss out on the joy and fulfillment that can be ours today. Another danger is that people can fear a particular event to the extent that they begin to expect that it will happen, thus causing it to happen. Psychologists explain this phenomena by saying that we move in the direction of our most dominant thought.

The birds of happiness and the birds of unhappiness are all around us. Which group will you invite to build a nest in your hair? When frightening thoughts enter the consciousness, we can choose what to do with them. One of the best ways I know of sending them on their way is to replace them with life-affirming thoughts. I focus on hope and all the values that keep me motivated to manage diabetes well.

Health and cheerfulness mutually beget each other.
–Joseph Addison

What are your values that motivate you to take up the daily challenges involved with the management of diabetes? Although I can readily tick off the values in my life (such as love for family, desire to have the energy to do my work well, the very basic desire to feel well), I appreciate holding in my heart more poetic expressions of those values. Because I do not consider myself poetic, I am always appreciative of those who are.

Such a poet was a soldier in the Persian Gulf. His lovely, thought-provoking comment was: "I'm ready to fight . . . but I'm here for the sunsets."

My thought in response to his comment was: "Aren't we all?"

Although I do not like the metaphor of war/violence/fighting, I know that I'm ready to take on whatever challenge that I must. However, I'm not looking for struggles to overcome. I'm looking for beautiful sunsets to enjoy.

That's the poetic reason that I poke my fingers, take insulin, eat nutritiously, and exercise regularly.

I love sunsets.

Difficulties strengthen the mind, as labor does the body.

—Seneca

"Into each life some rain must fall," Henry Wadsworth Longfellow pointed out to us in his poem *The Rainy Day*. As I read meditatively, I ask questions such as: What do you mean by rain? Is it a sprinkle? A gentle, steady rain? Heavy winds and hail? A hurricane? A light rain brings moisture to make flowers bloom and grass grow. Heavy winds, hail, and, certainly, a hurricane will do devastating damage.

So, what was Longfellow trying to say? Is he telling me that rain must fall so that grass and flowers can grow? Or is he saying that rain, symbolic of life's challenges and trials, is part of everyone's life? For me the poem says that life has challenges and problems and their presence in our lives helps us learn to cope and problem solve. Their presence helps us to appreciate the sun ever the more because we have known darkness.

In Robert Fulghum's book *Uh-Oh: Some Observations from Both Sides of the Refrigerator Door*, we hear that life is lumpy. "But, a lump in the oatmeal, a lump in the throat, and a lump in the breast are not the same lump."

That's the sort of discernment that I need when I consider the rain that falls in my life. I hope that I can be philosophical about the smaller problems. "Some rain" is good for my garden, and challenges help me grow.

Look not mournfully into the Past. It comes not back again. Wisely improve the Present. It is thine. Go forth to meet the shadowy Future, without fear.
—Henry Wadsworth Longfellow

Sometimes we create our own winters of despair. Overindulgence in food is perhaps the most common challenge for people with diabetes. People who have an alcohol problem can give up alcohol completely. People with diabetes have to continue to eat. Many people with diabetes actually plan for an occasional overindulgence and "weather" the experience well.

Many people, however, report that they are filled with remorse, regret, and guilt following an experience of overeating. Because thoughts create feelings, one might speculate that the thoughts in this instance would include shame, self-criticism, and hopelessness. These thoughts can lead to more overeating when people just give up and stop trying to get back in control of their lives.

Let us approach these times of winter with compassion for ourselves. Now is the moment to take action. Let the past go.

One woman's ingenious response to the prospect of chemotherapy helped to make the entire experience manageable . . . even beautifully meaningful.

The woman facing chemotherapy wrote to her adult children and to her closest friends. She asked them to send her something that was meaningful to them. She also asked for the story . . . the meaning in the object. Her plan was to return each object to its owner after she had taken it with her to her chemotherapy sessions. She viewed this plan as a way to keep herself distracted from the chemotherapy session and to remind herself of all her loved ones—her reason for wanting to live.

It worked better than she could have predicted. At each appointment, she set out all of the treasures sent by friends and family. As she set each one down, she told the story behind it. Sometimes a member of her family or a friend was with her at her appointments. The nurse administering the drugs got so involved in this activity that sometimes she would start telling the story behind one of the treasures to the guest.

The woman had wanted the items to remind her of her loved ones. She didn't realize how loved she would feel as she looked at the treasures surrounding her.

Help me to feel the love that is all around me.

Sunshine is delicious, rain is refreshing, wind braces up, snow is exhilarating; there is no such thing as bad weather, only different kinds of good weather.

–John Ruskin

Retirement is sometimes viewed as a negative time in life's cycles. The "productive years" (whatever that means!) are thought to be over, and people slow down. Other people view retirement as the time for engaging in all the fun activities that were put on the back burner during the hectic, busy work years. It seems, however, that retirement—like life—is what you make it.

A woman who had looked forward to retirement was surprised to find that once she retired, she found life dull and boring. She lost the feeling of energy that she had during her working years. She no longer had something to look forward to on a daily basis.

Then she discovered what she considers an exciting and meaningful project. She collects various flowers and weeds, presses them, arranges them into attractive works of art, and frames them. In the Spring, Summer, and Fall, she collects her raw materials. In the Winter she dries, arranges, and frames them to sell at craft fairs.

This seemingly small and simple change in her life has had an enormous impact on her attitude. Once again she is excited, enthusiastic, and happy. She would tell you that there are no bad seasons in life, only different kinds of seasons.

Retirement is the summer joy of finding things you like to do, the fall wisdom to do them, the winter courage to try new things, and the spring faith to keep saying "Yes."

God, grant me serenity to accept the things
I cannot change, courage to change the things
I can, and wisdom to know the difference.
                                    –Reinhold Niebuhr

Niebuhr's *Serenity Prayer* is world famous for the sense that it makes and the inspiration that it gives. Many of us are aware of this prayer, and yet we forget, we get busy, we don't pause to reflect. It is only through our reflection, our inward journey, that we remain aware of our vast resources. If we have known serenity at any point in our life, then serenity is one of our resources . . . however deeply buried it may be.

Something like the loss of a job can make people feel "backed into a corner." They have to do something next, but worry consumes them. When they are able to let go of the worry, they can experience the serenity that will help them take the next step and the next—the serenity of which Niebuhr wrote.

Think of a time when you felt a total calm that could be described with the word, "serenity." Close your eyes and recapture that moment. Then, apply that serenity to something in your life that you cannot change. Has diabetes backed you into a corner? Or do you have serenity in your corner backing you up?

Continuing to think about Niebuhr's *Serenity Prayer*, consider what memories come to you when you think of courage. I remember being a skinny 12-year-old about to do my first abdominal injection of insulin. I didn't want to do it. That was back in the days when we used steel needles and glass syringes. Shots were painful, and I did not want to push one of those "nails" into my tender midsection.

No less than two doctors coached me. I finally pushed the needle into the pinch of skin, only to have it come right out the other side of the pinch. I quickly glanced up to catch the most horrified expressions on the faces of the doctors. Suddenly, I felt very brave.

Every experience we have ever had with courage becomes a resource for us in the future. Courage begets courage. It builds upon itself.

When you reread a classic, you do not see more in the book than you did before; you see more in you than there was before.
                                   –Clifton Fadiman

The third spiritual quality in Niebuhr's prayer is wisdom. And it is wisdom that keeps us returning to the well of our inner resources to draw on the past experiences, the lessons learned, the dreams yet to be realized, and the faith that we really do have all the resources we will ever need.

Inspiration and intuition team up to connect our plain, everyday experiences to the wisdom that lies deep within us. When this happens, we typically have one of those Aha! moments. When the staff of a clinic in Wisconsin invited me to speak at their annual meeting, I asked whether they had a theme. They told me: The Wizard of Oz. This Aha! immediately connected me with the SERENITY (heart) of Tin Man, the COURAGE of Lion, and the WISDOM (brains) of Scarecrow.

I enjoyed the movie *The Wizard of Oz* when I was a child. I keep enjoying it year after year. I continue to marvel at how much meaning this adventure film has. The quote helped me to understand how this could be.

*T*he *Wizard of Oz* provides many rich metaphors. The Wizard himself is a metaphor for the magic bullet—the sure cure that so many of us seek, convinced that an answer to our questions exists outside of us. But, ultimately, he was a scam artist. He used Dorothy and her friends to get rid of the Wicked Witch of the West but did not—because he could not—deliver on his promise to return Dorothy and Toto to Kansas.

Dorothy herself had the power to return to Kansas. She had the ruby red slippers and the mantra, "There's no place like home." Lyrics to the song "Tin Man" by the band America reinforce the idea that answers are found inside of us, not outside. Each of us has the wisdom we need.

Oz never did give nothin' to the Tin Man that he didn't, didn't already have.

The charm and happy outcome of the Wizard's scam tactics of putting requests back on the people doing the asking, resulted in their empowerment—they discovered their own resources.

What resource have you been seeking?
Look inside.

One of today's trendy terms is intentional living. This term is used to describe a "take charge" sort of approach to life. Rather than mindlessly following cultural dictates about behavior, people are encouraged to think about their life and make conscious choices about how they will live it.

Consider trying intentional listening. Each of us has a treasury of wisdom deep inside. When does your wisdom bubble up from your soul to reach your conscious mind? While reading a book or article that takes you beneath the surface of life? Following a tragedy or other profound life experience that defies reason and rationality?

With intentional listening, we are proactive instead of reactive. Rather than waiting for a life event to call forth our wisdom, we seek it. Here are two ways to do this. One is to gather a group of people for a discussion. A book is commonly the focal point for group discussion. Intentional listening is practiced as each person who speaks is given the group's full attention. The other way to engage in intentional listening is to ask profound questions during meditation. Alone in a place where you will not be disturbed and free from a "deadline" for completing your meditation, you listen first for the questions that are already in your soul. Then you ask questions of your own. These questions may be:

What is diabetes trying to teach me?

How can I use my experience with diabetes for growth?

How do I define quality of life? How does diabetes fit into that definition?

When a friend of mine who is characteristically optimistic and upbeat was depressed, he told me that he actually welcomes feeling "down." He explained that these depressions don't last. The lesson they bring is that they make him aware of feeling. "I am grateful that I can feel," he told me. "I may not celebrate feeling down the way I celebrate joy, but both joy and despair are needed to make me whole."

Help me to sense my wholeness
when I am hurting.

Remember how you feel when an irritating noise, flashing light, or body ache suddenly stops? Perhaps you experience a calm, relaxed state. Awareness of that calm is similar to "being present in the moment." This expression is used by people who engage in mindful meditation.

A calm, relaxed state is best for spiritual communication. The "still, small voice within" can be heard better when outside distractions are at a minimum and when inner turmoil is quieted.

A psychologist friend said he recommends to clients that they close their eyes and imagine a large gunnysack outside the room in which they choose to meditate. He suggests that people identify concerns and, one by one, drop them into the sack where they can be retrieved later. Our concerns need to be dealt with, but meditation requires a quiet mind, a peaceful soul.

Pour calm into my mind and peace into my heart as I seek your wisdom.

Just to be is a blessing.
Just to live is holy.

–Rabbi Abraham Heschel

When we have nothing, we learn a lot about ourselves . . . and about life. We learn what we value, what we really need, and who we really are. Without distractions like money, power, position (even a job), we can focus on what we do have. This is a crash course in values clarification.

Diabetes has the power to drive the same process.

Just when we feel we've been deprived of the "good" that life offers (desserts? the lifestyle of a couch potato?), we realize that the promise of the good life is an empty promise, and we re-evaluate the meaning of "good life."

What is included in your definition of the good life? Are there values and beliefs that you live by? Are there simple pleasures that delight you? Are you engaged in meaningful work (volunteer or otherwise)? Do you give of yourself to help others?

A father who had lost his 14-month-old son to heart disease commented that there is no getting over the loss of a child but that a "new normal" evolves. In this new normal, there can be laughter and joy. He had not believed that normal joy could be part of his life anymore. He said that working on a charity event to raise money for the local children's hospital made his new normal brighter.

After a while, life with a chronic disease evolves to a new normal.

Diabetes can be viewed initially as a series of losses: the loss of the former self, the loss of the previous lifestyle, the loss of a dream. However, a new normal evolves, and we can see our new self as stronger, our new lifestyle as healthier, and new dreams emerge that can be more deeply meaningful and precious.

A dear friend of mine shared a story with me about her experience with kidney dialysis. Several times a week she had to be hooked up to a dialysis machine. To say it was a task she did not enjoy would be a great understatement. My friend struggled with her feelings—gratitude that she could be kept alive through dialysis, yet resentful of this largely unpleasant experience that took her away from meaningful activity.

One day the nurse who worked with her told my friend that she was studying to become a naturalized citizen of the United States. From that time on, whenever my friend had dialysis, she quizzed the nurse about American policy and citizenship. The time passed quickly, and my friend experienced the great reward of knowing that she was helping someone.

All the world's a stage.

—William Shakespeare

Shakespeare said that we are actors on the world's stage. We play many roles. "Diabetic" does not describe who I am, but I believe that word does describe one of the roles I play in life.

In the theatre, actors play their roles only when they step onto a physical stage. In life, we are "on stage" every moment of every day. We play numerous roles at the same time, but always we play our diabetic role.

There are certain roles that I enjoy more than others. I like my roles as wife, mother, and educator. Actually, it is because of the roles I enjoy that I work at doing the diabetes role well. I want to continue enjoying my current roles, and I want to be healthy so that I can experience the future role of a happy, healthy retiree.

I don't expect an Academy Award for the way I've played my roles. Please help me to play my roles to the best of my ability.

Because health care professionals may read this book, I write this message to them and, of course, to people with diabetes because we work with health care professionals as part of a team.

In the book *Gung Ho* by Kenneth Blanchard and Sheldon Bowles, I read a marvelous analogy. "Running a business from numbers is like playing basketball while watching the scoreboard instead of the ball." Eureka! I immediately saw the application in diabetes. Managing diabetes by focusing on blood glucose numbers reduces diabetes self-management to a numbers game and ignores the bigger picture—the game of life and the person who is playing it.

Blanchard and Bowles advise business people to look after the basics if they want success, and the first *basic* is the person. Is the person happy? It's the same in diabetes. Is the person enjoying life? Is the person experiencing a (self-defined) fulfilling life? Is the person coping well?

How is the *person*? When the *person* is doing well, the numbers will reflect that.

Help us to work together.
Help us all to see the big picture.

I often hear people say that having diabetes in and of itself is not so bad. What is tough are all the management tasks—daily, even hourly—carrying out the appropriate eating, exercising, and monitoring. Life with diabetes is a never-ending juggling act. And if, from time to time, one of the "balls" gets dropped, it is not because the juggler is *noncompliant*, that is, uncooperative. Balls get dropped because constant, never-ending juggling is tiring, tedious, and difficult.

**Grant me the energy to keep juggling . . .
and the wisdom to seek help when I need it.
And, give my "helpers" wisdom so that they
can help me and not judge me.**

Eleanor's story is a story of love, courage, wisdom, and faith. Eleanor is my mother. I have told this story on three continents to thousands of people. I include it here, in case you have never heard it.

I was diagnosed with diabetes in 1957 just ten months after my father died unexpectedly. Mother was a 39-year-old widow with her second great challenge: a little girl with a chronic disease, diabetes. When I asked my mother what diabetes meant, she smiled and enthusiastically told me:

Diabetes means that we are going to learn so much about good nutrition. It means that we're going to live such a healthy lifestyle, the whole family will benefit because you have diabetes. And you will always be a stronger, more self-disciplined person because you have diabetes.

She set me on a healthy path. The positive attitude that she presented to me gave me strength to cope with diabetes. Nineteen years later I drew strength from what she taught me to help our son when he was seriously injured at birth. Before we knew the lasting impact of his injury, I *knew* it would make him strong. Her legacy is one of love and wisdom and faith.

Thank you, Eleanor.

Wisdom is a tree of life to those who embrace her;
happy are those who hold her tightly.

–Proverbs 3:18

The diagnosis of a chronic disease can cast a shadow over the future. People sometimes respond to their diagnosis by putting future plans on hold.

As I write this book, we are approaching the year 2000. I am aware that people historically (or hysterically?) view a new millennium as potentially the end of the world. Fearful questions arise.

One of our pastors gave a sermon on the new millennium. His conclusion was: It's time to plant a tree.

When I was diagnosed with diabetes as a child, people in our small community commented to one another that I would not live to be 21 years old. Forty-one years after diagnosis, I am enjoying the fruits of a healthy life. I'm grateful that my mother planted a tree . . . the tree of life.

Help me to look to the future
with joyful anticipation and faith.

Resiliency is an important quality in all of life. We frequently observe it in nature. I have seen robins rebuild their nests after their first was demolished by an April blizzard. Flowers beaten flat to the ground by wind and driving rain find their way to stand up again with the return of gentler breezes and sunshine.

There is a spirit of resiliency in the human soul that amazes some, escapes others, and inspires those who are willing to invest in it. Diabetes is filled with examples because living positively with diabetes requires that people be resilient.

Unlike infections that can be cured and broken bones that can be fixed, diabetes does not go away. Neither is it easily managed. Many variables in life affect blood glucose levels from hormones to stress to failed therapeutic interventions. If only we could "quit" diabetes the way we can quit a job for which we feel ill-suited. But we can't. So, we make a decision about that in which we will "invest."

What is the return on an investment in self-pity?

What is the return on an investment in blame, denial, or anger?

I see resiliency as the process of investing in such "blue chip stocks" as courage, faith, joy, and wisdom. The return on that investment is a richer, fuller life, including living positively with diabetes . . . or any challenge.

Far away, there in the sunshine are my highest aspirations. I may not reach them, but I can look up and see them and try to follow where they lead.

–Louisa May Alcott

The greatest challenges of life are those that give us the opportunity to transcend (rise above, overcome) pain. When we overcome our pain, we are immediately connected to an elite of humankind, people who have also risen above pain. There are many. Here are a few statements from some of these special people:

The marvelous richness of human experience would lose something of rewarding joy if there were no limitations to overcome. The hilltop hour would not be so wonderful if there were no dark valleys to traverse.

–Helen Keller

I have learned that success is to be measured not so much by the position that one has reached in life, as by the obstacles which one has overcome while trying to succeed.

–Booker T. Washington

You can't help getting older, but you don't have to get old.

–George Burns

The artists of life—poets, painters, musicians, playwrights, and novelists—give us insights into how we go about transcending pain. Being artists they, of course, give their "advice" in language that causes us to search our hearts, where each of us finds our own insights.

Rituals help to give us ways to address life events, giving the events meaning and the rituals purpose. In the early 1970s, our nation was dealing with the aftermath of the Vietnam war. To lend support, many people wore the names of soldiers missing in action around their wrists. The intent of these people was to continue wearing the ID bracelet until the soldier was found.

It was 1976 when our baby was born . . . and seriously injured because of a hospital mistake. He needed to remain hospitalized after I was released. When I left the hospital, I cut the plastic hospital ID off my wrist, but I left the second hospital ID on . . . it was John's.

For weeks I went to the hospital each day and spent the entire day there, nursing, bathing, enjoying my baby. At night I returned home.

Twenty-seven days after John was born, we brought him home. That evening as my husband and I sat at the kitchen table having dinner, I took the kitchen shears and, with neither fanfare nor ceremony, quietly cut the ID from my wrist. Our little MIA was home at last.

With all the heartache and concern over John's injury, I had been helped with this simple gesture of wearing his ID. I felt connected to the many people whose concerns were similar though far greater. I drew on their strength. I hope they received some of mine.

Joseph Campbell studied heroes from ancient literature, including the Bible and Greek mythology. He saw similarities and identified what he referred to as the Hero's Journey. He said that all such journeys begin with a call to adventure. This call could be a compelling invitation to great danger, not necessarily an "adventure" such as skiing the Rockies. Campbell was a consultant on the Star Wars movies. Luke Skywalker received a harrowing call to adventure!

All of us receive calls to adventure throughout our lifetime. When we receive a call, we make a monumental, life-transforming choice. To say "no" is to admit defeat and give up. But, to say "yes" we take on enormous challenges, problems, discomfort, and uncertainties. The reward, if we "make it," is a transformation of our life.

Campbell pointed out the huge dilemma that the human race faces. We want to have the strength without the hard work. We want to be heroic but not have to suffer. But, the growth comes as we travel through pain. It is our trials that transform us.

When diabetes enters our lives, we are called to an adventure. We can refuse to answer the call, at great risk to our health and well-being. Or we can choose to accept the call with all the challenges and problems inherent in it.

Another trait of the Hero's Journey is that the hero has an advisor who helps guide him through the "snakes" and "dragons" along the way. The advisor for those of us who have diabetes is the diabetes health care team.

Don't leave on your journey without them.

The lack of knowledge is darker than the night.

–African saying

The mother of a friend of mine was diagnosed with diabetes. I was quite young and made the assumption that my friend's mother was making the same lifestyle changes that I was, learning much of the same information for living well with diabetes.

Many years later, I returned to my hometown for a funeral. I was surprised when I saw my friend's mother and realized that she had had a leg amputated. I was stunned when I heard her ask, as sandwiches were being passed to her, "Is there any sugar in these?"

She had never learned the basics about diabetes. She didn't know about food being converted into glucose. What happened?

Let each of us serve to guide people to the American Diabetes Association, to a diabetes educator, to education—the beacon of light that is life.

If you surrender to the wind, you can ride it.
                                    —Toni Morrison

Surrender is very difficult for most of us to do. We want to be in control. But when we feel in need of help, the idea of surrender becomes appealing . . . if we feel trust and faith in the person or entity to which we surrender.

When we were very small children, the fortunate among us had parents who were worthy of our trust . . . people to whom we could surrender when we were "getting in over our heads." That's why I like the image of God as a Heavenly Father . . . completely worthy of my trust.

In a physical application of surrender, I think of the times when my diabetes has soared dangerously out of control. I am so grateful to have had a doctor whom I trust and into whose care I could surrender and feel at peace.

Surrender to the wind symbolizes the ultimate spiritual act: trusting the unseen. If the wind symbolizes the spirit, what would it mean to you to ride it? I can imagine being taken through the tree tops, into a bird's nest, and landing gently on a flower petal. I try to imagine the myriad places that this wind could take me.

I surrender.

Stories of how other people have courageously overcome their difficulties are a great source of inspiration. We all seek to celebrate a triumph of the human spirit.

Marilyn Hamilton fell from a hang glider and ended up paralyzed from the waist down. She complained one day to her hang-gliding friends that wheelchairs were like steel dinosaurs: heavy, awkward, and ugly. They got together to design a wheelchair using the lightweight metal used for hang gliders.

The result was the Quickie wheelchair . . . and a successful new business venture. Marilyn designed the wheelchairs to have vibrant colors. She says: "If you can't stand up, stand out."

That is spirit. Her story is a triumph and an inspiration.

People who inspire us can be (and often are) an ongoing source of inspiration. My mother has been.

One Thanksgiving she invited our entire extended family: my married sisters' in-laws, the aunts, uncles, and cousins . . . lots of people. Because I live out of town, I couldn't be there to help with anything except the last minute details.

Concerned for my mother, I asked her, "Why do you work so hard?"

With joy in her face, she responded: "Because I'm so thankful that I can."

I thought of the gentleman from Washington whose Pappy had advised him to have an attitude of gratitude. My mother's life is an expression of that attitude.

Who are the beams of light in your life?

Laughter is the sun that drives winter from the human face.

−Victor Hugo

Ancient wisdom supports the idea that laughter is good medicine. Legendary comedian Milton Berle said, "Laughter is an instant vacation." That wisdom is made real in the life of a friend of mine who rents funny movies when he is feeling down and wants to get back up.

I think of what a gift this particular friend is to me because he loves to laugh, and he laughs a lot. When he laughs, he lifts all of us who are with him. We can see the sun in his face and feel its warmth in our hearts.

I cherish my friends who make me laugh. Thanks, Mike.

P.S. Reminder: Because winter has such short days and long nights, it is a good season for seeing funny movies or reading funny books. I laughed so hard when I read the essay on the mother of the bride in a Robert Fulghum book that I cried . . . which was a little embarrassing because I was sitting alone on an airplane.

Every tomorrow has two handles. We can take hold of it with the handle of anxiety or the handle of faith.

–H.W. Beecher

Anxiety is common to all of us. We've explored a bit of the anxiety-provoking aspects of life in the Winter section of this book. Now it is time to enter into Spring and explore faith. Beecher's comment makes it seem as though we have simply to choose between anxiety and faith. But grasping hold of the handle of faith is not easy, it is not a "simple" choice.

In fact, it is a choice that we make many times, through many tomorrows. How often have I chosen to have faith, to let go and let God, only to find myself wrestling back the control for anxieties that I really want no part of? Life is very ironic at times.

Let us explore our choices . . . again. Let us choose life.

Life is either a daring adventure or nothing.
Security does not exist in nature, nor do the
children of men as a whole experience it.
Avoiding danger is no safer in the long run than
exposure.

–Helen Keller

This quotation brings to mind an image of covered wagons rumbling across the plains. People moving with all their belongings to a place they've never been . . . places no one's been. For most of us, "daring adventure" is a term that invites thoughts of physical challenges—biking across the state, scaling tall mountains, or swimming the English Channel.

But by the courageous, enthusiastic way Helen Keller lived her life, despite being blind and deaf, she demands that we take a deeper look at what we call a "daring adventure." Blindness makes an adventure out of the seemingly simplest tasks, like getting dressed or cooking a meal. One of my dearest friends is blind due to diabetes. Though she cannot see, she has remarkable "vision" that takes her on unlimited adventures. Taken inwardly, her adventures produce insights that enrich her life and all who know her.

Whatever the destination on a daring adventure, we have to face our fears of the unknown. We have to go inside to find the courage it takes—whether we are changing careers, taking the trip of a lifetime, injecting insulin, or writing a difficult letter to a friend.

The greatest, most daring adventures are those we take into totally uncharted areas. What have your most daring adventures been—physically, emotionally, mentally, spiritually? Have you ever had the experience of slipping your hand into God's and saying, "Yes. Whatever—wherever. Count me in."

Tell someone about one of your daring adventures. Think about your next one.

Spring

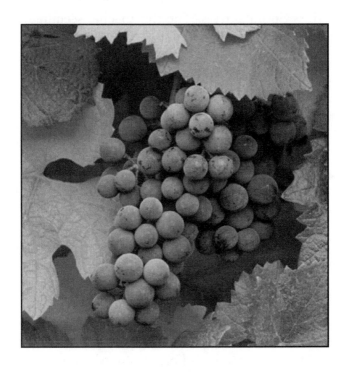

Introduction to Spring

*The most beautiful thing we can experience is
the mystery.*

                                    –Albert Einstein

Near the end of each winter when I have looked
so long at the frozen world, I begin to think about
the mystery and miracle that we will experience
when Spring arrives. The sun touches seemingly
dead branches, and the tree responds with its
"Yes!" to life. It sends forth a tiny bud, containing
a green leaf that startles me each year with its
freshness, its lacy beauty, its remarkable "spirit." It
never fails to awaken and inspire my spirit, too.
The mystery of life—how does it happen? Again,
the physical season mimics the spiritual—or is it
the spiritual that mimics the physical? Spring's
story is one of Faith and Hope.

Healing stories offer hope. All of us have hurts.
Many of us experience tragedy, and there is no
"getting over" tragic events in our lives. They
become part of our story, part of who we are and
always will be. So, we are never healed from deep
hurts, but we can actively seek healing—which on
the soul level may be acceptance of what has happened and love of who we are now. The miracle
is that we can be whole again when we are

engaged in the healing process. I have participated in my own healing story and have heard the healing stories of many people. Some have nothing to do with diabetes but everything to do with the human dimension of hurting, finding hope, and healing. I believe that when we stop healing, we start hurting. The miracle is in the process, because healing is always available to us. When we choose to seek healing, it is the flame of Hope that illuminates our way.

In this section, we explore some faith traditions because these are often the bridges we take to connect our hope with our faith. The voices you hear include: Jesse Jackson, Elizabeth Kübler-Ross, Albert Einstein, African and Russian proverbs, the Bible, the Torah, and American Indian philosophy. From India come painted prayers and the faith of Mother Teresa. All of these voices are shared to help you connect with the faith that resides uniquely in your soul.

In a deeply spiritual sense, we are all involved in what Thoreau referred to as "the art of living" through which we each affect the quality of the day—for ourselves, for those around us, for all humankind. I have faith and evidence that this is so.

Whatever the source of your faith, may you reconnect with it as you read the Spring section. May the blessing of true well-being be yours.

When I was nine years old, my father died unexpectedly of a heart attack. Three weeks after I turned ten, I was diagnosed with diabetes. These significant life events inspired some deep thinking that may be uncharacteristic of children that age. Although I still thought about childhood games and goals, I asked questions about the meaning of life . . . questions more commonly addressed in middle age.

I remember a prayer that I said every night:

> *I do not ask a truce*
> *With life's incessant pain,*
> *But school my lips, Lord,*
> *Not to complain.*
>
> *I do not ask for peace*
> *From life's constant sorrow,*
> *But, give me the courage, Lord,*
> *To face tomorrow.*

The prayer never struck me as being either morbid or sad. The prayer helped me to feel strong, by connecting me to the source of my strength. At the age of ten, I was a wise little old lady. I knew that life was tough . . . and, still, joyful.

People are like stained glass windows; they sparkle and shine when the sun is out, but when the darkness sets in, their true beauty is revealed only if there is a Light within.

—Elizabeth Kübler-Ross

Poets, philosophers, and theologians talk about the importance of inner light to illuminate the spiritual path. That thought points to the reason that people engage in self-reflection: to explore and define the source of that inner light, the mysterious but ever-present Light within.

Help me to keep my inner light lit.

Where there is hope there is life, where there is life there is possibility, and where there is possibility change can occur.

—Jesse Jackson

People with diabetes are asked to make lifestyle changes. Sometimes these changes are significantly different from their current lifestyle. Before change can occur physically, mental and spiritual work must be done.

We can change our thinking so that we view lifestyle change as positive or, at least, tolerable. THERE IS HOPE. Health care professionals can teach us the skills we need to manage diabetes and participate actively in life. THERE IS POSSIBILITY. By connecting with our source of faith, we lay a foundation of

HOPE on which we build that changed and healthy life.

Help me to maintain HOPE, that I might have Life with all its POSSIBILITIES.

Imagination is more important than knowledge because knowledge is limited.
                                        –Albert Einstein

Nearly 20 years ago, an endocrinologist looked into my eyes and said, "You can expect to require treatment within the year." Although I am aware of and grateful for laser treatments for retinopathy, I had never required treatment before and wasn't willing to simply accept the fact that I would require it. I had no "plan" except to have faith and remain open.

Just weeks later I attended a class entitled "Creative Visualization and Mental Imagery." The lecturer told us that the mind can heal the body when we visualize the "hurting" part as healed... not healing, but healed and whole.

As I listened, many thoughts went through my mind: imagery, imagination, mind/body connections . . . I made the decision to use mental imagery and to visualize my retinas as perfectly healthy, with no microaneurysms. I found a photograph of a healthy retina in a magazine. I cut it out and taped it onto the inside of a door in my office. I memorized it.

At my next appointment, my endocrinologist told me that the microaneurysms were gone. How is that explained?

Blood glucose monitoring had just been introduced. Glycated hemoglobin results provided a treatment benchmark. Perhaps it is because I had better tools for self-management that I have never developed serious eye disease. Perhaps it is because there is a mind/body connection . . . that I tapped into.

Perhaps . . .

Laura's Garden is a place of beauty, healing, love, and hope. The garden commemorates the life and light of a little girl who died following a horse-riding accident. The garden, located at Laura's elementary school, was built by her family, her school friends (including the principal and teachers), and a community seeking healing and meaning.

At the program to officially recognize Laura's garden, her pastor spoke. He said, "The question is not *where* is God? The question is *when* is God? The when is now." We saw God's hand and Laura's spirit in:

- Statements of love from her parents, sister, and aunt
- A poem read by a family friend
- A song written from Laura's perspective, thanking people for taking care of her garden
- Essays written by classmates, read by the school's social worker
- The large group of children and adults gathered to celebrate Laura and her garden
- The trees, plants, flowers, waterfall, pond, and bridge
- The tiny, new butterflies released from boxes at the end of the ceremony

I will return to Laura's Garden whenever I need the healing it offers to those who have lost loved ones. I will remember my father, my nephew, my son's college roommate, aunts, uncles, and friends. I will see them in the beauty of all living things. I will thank God for their lives and Laura's.

In the late 1980s, I served on the board of governors of an inner city hospital in Minneapolis. Because of the very challenging health care environment, we made the decision to merge with another downtown hospital, hoping that we could be financially stronger together. The interesting part of the merger is that we merged a Christian hospital and a Jewish hospital.

To ensure that everyone in our new hospital would feel nurtured, the board mandated a Spiritual Focus Committee. I had the privilege to chair it. We all felt blessed by this experience as we learned about one another's traditions and worked together for our patients, our hospital, and our community.

At the dedication of our All-Faiths Chapel, a Christian chaplain and a Jewish rabbi officiated. The rabbi gave the benediction. He said: "May we continue to respect our differences and love what we share." As is true of great truths, that statement has universal applications, one of which is world peace.

Because that statement was seared in my soul, I saw another application—in chronic disease. There is a "community" of people with chronic diseases. There are differences; that is, some have arthritis, lupus, asthma, heart disease, or diabetes. Our challenges may be different, but we share the life-affirming spiritual values of love, hope, peace, wisdom, and joy.

Help us to share what we love.

Hope is the pillar of the world.

HOPE is the very cornerstone of life. But for some, hope can be wishful thinking. People can hope for things, experiences, outcomes. Hope in this context is a verb. For others, hope can be the faith upon which the foundation of their life is built. They have hope, no matter what things, experiences, or outcomes are present in their lives. Hope in this context is a noun.

How do you use the word hope? Reflect on how much wishful thinking you do. Listen for the word hope when you speak. What evidence do you find that hope is the foundation of your life?

Are you hoping for a good life or do you have hope that you will?

Great art hangs in museums. Great art is heard in concert halls and celebrated in theatres. There is, in addition, a great art that resides within each of us. Henry David Thoreau called it the highest of arts: the art of living.

People who practice this art are not artists in the usual sense. They are people who, through the nobility of their lives, have affected what Thoreau called the "quality" of the day.

We can affect the quality of the day for ourselves and others . . . turning dark to light . . . fear to courage . . . frustration to patience . . . loneliness to joy. Our words are music just as surely as our lives paint a picture. From our hearts, through our words and actions, we create the beauty of kindness, patience, harmony, and hope.

When I see someone engaged in an act of kindness, I am watching a great artist creating a masterpiece, affecting the quality of the day for everyone.

A kind word is like a Spring day.

–Russian proverb

Soul-er power is what it will take to change our paradigm.

–Martin J. Sullivan, MD.
Director, Healing the Heart Program
Duke University Medical Center

Health care professionals talk a lot about the "new paradigm" (model). They recognize that the medical model for acute care does not adequately address the needs of people with chronic diseases. In the medical model, the disease is taken care of (treated or "fixed") by medical professionals. But, diabetes needs "care" on a daily—even hourly—basis when medical professionals are not there to provide it.

Diabetes is managed by the person who has it with the advice and support of a health care team. For this model to work, everyone must understand that the person with diabetes is a whole person: body, mind, and spirit.

Let us all consider the notion of soul-er power. What is it? How do we harness it? How can health care professionals nourish it in their patients? How can we who have diabetes nurture and tap into it?

As I encouraged you in the Winter section of this book, I invite you to read meditatively and consider . . . what is soul-er power?

Choice is a critical aspect of living well with challenges like diabetes. We choose our behaviors and our attitudes. We choose how responsibly we will take action on the information we get from our health care team and from daily blood glucose monitoring. We choose the thoughts that will help to make diabetes self-management an onerous burden or an opportunity for good health and personal growth.

I have a poster in my office that reminds me of the most basic choice of all, the choice of life itself. Reflect on your choices and on these words:

Before you this day there is set good and evil, life and death . . . . Choose life.
–Deuteronomy 30:19

In late March of 1998, a tornado ravaged southern Minnesota. More than a mile wide, the tornado uprooted trees and shattered homes into splinters.

My friend and mentor, Robert Esbjornson, lost nearly everything. His computer was sucked into the angry sky. A treasured painting was stolen by the unrelenting force of the wind. His bed was reduced to its metal frame. Momentos of a 45-year marriage—gone. The arboretum in front of his picture window was now treeless.

As he walked through the rubble and surveyed the damage and devastation, he said he could hear a sort of music in his head. When he paused to listen, he realized that he was hearing bits of Psalms going through his head. A habit of reading a Psalm each day was providing him with strength, peace, and comfort.

When I thought, 'My foot slips,' thy steadfast love, O Lord, held me up.
When the cares of my heart are many, thy consolations cheer my soul.

—Psalm 94:18,19

It is wise to furnish one's mind well. When it's all you have left, you want a rich treasury.

May the Footprints we leave behind
Show that we've walked in Kindness
Toward the earth and every living thing.

This lovely thought was inspired by American Indian philosophy. It is an example of how we can transcend or rise above the many, momentary problems of daily life.

Some days we get so concerned about dusty footprints on a newly waxed floor that we miss the bigger picture . . . of life. Pause today to see above the daily challenges and ponder the footprints you are leaving.

Help me to transcend my frustrations
with diabetes and all its tasks.
Help me to walk in kindness.

One Sunday morning as I listened to the children in our Sunday School program sing, I received the gift of an awakening to a new thought. The children were moving their hands through the air as if their hands were boats going through waves. The words to the song were: "With Christ in my vessel, I can smile at the storm." In that very instant, I saw vessels to mean blood vessels, not boats. I experienced a peace that told me no matter what the future holds, I don't need to worry.

I cannot possibly know the details of what that means. I can't "know" that I will never develop blood vessel complications. But, at a far deeper level of understanding and life, I can and I do know that I will be fine. What amazing peace there is in that.

*All my life through, the new sights of Nature
made me rejoice like a child.*

–Marie Curie

Spring has a magical beauty that inspires thoughts of new beginnings. The lacy, light, yet brilliant green of new leaves is a thrilling sight each year. The earth's agenda to bring about new life inspires me to examine what I am doing to rejuvenate my life.

I will busy myself, along with Mother Earth, at the tasks of life. What the earth does naturally, she has reminded me to do intentionally—self-care. I will *re*-commit to the goals of good nutrition and invigorating exercise. I will take my "meds" (medications) and I will do my "meds" (meditations).

In mindfully attending to the health of my body, mind, and spirit, I am engaged in true self-care. The Earth and I are one.

Exposure to beauty can awaken the memory of beauty that resides in the soul. So, too, can hearing or reading wisdom awaken that quality within us. Consider the wisdom in this beautiful Talmudic saying:

Just as the hand held in front of the eye obscures the tallest of mountains, so can the stresses of everyday life keep us from seeing the awe, the wonder, and the mystery there is in the world.

What real or metaphoric "hand" might you have in front of your eyes? Name the stresses that currently obscure your vision.

What names can you give to the awe, wonder, and mystery that surround you?

Painted prayers are found in India where women are responsible for these visual petitions to the gods. Traditionally, these painted prayers ask for health and well-being.

Consider what your painted prayer would be. Instead of words, what would a prayer of pictures include? Would you have people in your picture? What would their faces look like if you were praying for spiritual qualities like peace, hope, joy, and love?

If you were praying for healing and wholeness, what symbols might you use in your painted prayer?

What colors would you choose? Red for enthusiasm, love, and compassion? Green for peace? Blue for wisdom? Yellow for joy?

Consider your painted prayer. Paint it if you have that gift. But at least, close your eyes and paint your prayer in your mind.

Work of sight is done. Now do heart work on the pictures within you.

–Rainer Maria Rilke

A United States senator reportedly interviewed Mother Teresa. He told her that no matter how hard she worked, millions of people would die. Her task was hopeless.

Mother Teresa's remarkable response was:

God does not require that I be successful. He asks that I be faithful.

Managing diabetes is not only a daily task, it requires hourly attention . . . if only a brief glance at one's watch to see when the next meal, monitoring, or exercise will occur.

The rewards most people seek include daily good health and the reasonable hope of avoiding serious long-term complications. There is a reward at a deeper level. It is *integrity of the spirit*. The very spirit that Mother Teresa spoke of.

You can experience integrity of the spirit when you follow healthy attitudes and behaviors at great cost with no guarantees of any reward. That's diabetes management. That's life.

Life is full of important tasks that we work at without being guaranteed the outcome we seek: parenting, marriage, jobs, friendships. Although there is no guarantee of success, there is a reasonable expectation that the harder we work, the better we will do. On my most frustrating days, however, when the blood sugars seem to defy my attempts at control, I realize that I may not be "successful," but I can be faithful.

Self-efficacy—the belief that we are capable—is regarded as one of the primary indicators that people will do well with a disease that requires self-management, a disease like diabetes. If people believe they can perform the tasks that manage their disease, they are more likely to perform them.

Whereas I do believe that, I also believe at a far deeper level that I need more than self-confidence. I need God confidence—the faith and belief that I am not alone.

And that He who is with me has the power to spin the galaxies. Such is my faith in God.

Trust in him at all times, O people; pour out your heart before him; God is a refuge for us.
—Psalm 62:8

Lo, I am with you always, to the close of the age.
—Matthew 28:20

Sometimes our light goes out
   but is blown into flame
by an encounter with another human being.
   Each of us owes the
   deepest thanks
to those who have kindled this inner light.
                              –Albert Schweitzer

We can have our inner lights kindled by people whom we know and by people whom we will never meet. We nourish hope by what we read and hear. Then, in moments of quiet reflection we reconnect with that wisdom.

Here are some of my favorites. What are yours?

In the depth of winter I finally realized that within me there lay an invincible summer.
                              –Albert Camus

We could never learn to be brave and patient if there were only joy in the world.
                              –Helen Keller

To give without any reward, or any notice, has a special quality of its own.
                              –Anne Morrow Lindbergh

The future belongs to those who believe in the beauty of their dreams.
                              –Eleanor Roosevelt

None are so old as those who have outlived enthusiasm.
                              –Henry David Thoreau

My son has been one of the single greatest sources of inspiration to me.

When he was born, an erroneous IV solution seriously burned him, taking away all the skin, fatty tissue, veins, and nerves from his knee to the middle of his foot. After two major plastic surgeries and a year of orthopedic devices, the medical world was done with their job by the time John turned four.

His healing and ours had only just begun. The horrendous scars on his leg received comment from children and adults. ("I've seen scars in my day, but what happened to you?!") We helped John to become "empowered" by developing his own response to both simple questions and rude ones.

When he was a junior in high school, he was getting his ankles taped in the training room before football practice. A young physician was saying to the boys, "I had four years of college after college to become a doctor!" Then, he noticed John's leg. He exclaimed, "What happened to you?"

John's modest response was, "Oh, some guy with four years of college after college made a mistake." I wish John had told the young physician about how we never sued. We all need to approach life with humility.

The day after the final football game of John's senior year, the entire team visited a children's hospital. John approached a little boy in a wheelchair, got on his knees so they could be eye-to-eye and said, "Tell me about you." The adoring little boy said, "I just love playin' baseball, but they say I won't walk the way I used to." In answer, John rolled up his pant leg as the little boy rolled up his pajama leg. The boys shared their scars, their stories, and their strength.

None of us will ever be quite the same.

David, the humble shepherd boy, conquered the evil giant, Goliath, using a slingshot and a well-placed smooth stone. Christians and Jews alike celebrate this Biblical hero.

David's single greatest attribute was his faith. He knew how small he was in comparison to Goliath. He surely would have felt more confident at the head of an army to stand with him against his foe. With no army and only a slingshot for a weapon, David relied upon the greatest power in the universe: God.

What are the "Goliaths" that you face in life? Is diabetes one of them? Or perhaps, several Goliaths lurk within this single disease?

How does faith play a role? It was faith that led David to pick up his slingshot and use it. If David's tool was a slingshot, then maybe our basic tool is a blood glucose meter. Diabetes can seem like such a huge obstacle that hopelessness becomes the real Goliath. It takes enormous faith to pick up our tools and use them.

Help me to receive faith. Help me to be faithful.

Abraham Lincoln wrote a father's reflection on his son's first day of school. As is true of all great literature, his words are equally appropriate for daughters, and, in fact, his thoughts are meaningful for us all.

Lincoln talks about his son embarking on a great adventure that "probably will include wars and tragedy and sorrow."

> To live in this world will require faith and love and courage. So World,
> teach him the things he will have to know.
> Teach him that it is far more honorable to fail than to cheat.
> Teach him to sell his brawn and his brains to the highest bidders, but never to put a price tag on his heart and soul.

These are inspiring words at any time. They were particularly significant for me and my family on the day we celebrated John's baptism. These thoughts helped to lift us above the pain and uncertainty of his injury to focus on what we really value. We were able to begin to understand that there is more to a child's life and future than an injury to his foot and leg.

Years later, I shared that thought with a group of children with diabetes and their parents. I suggested that we need to step back and see the whole picture and realize that there is more to life than diabetes. How interesting, though, that it is the diabetes or injury that calls forth the faith, love, and courage.

Is that what is meant by "a blessing in disguise?"

Another John story. When John was six years old, he came running to the front door to tell me that a baby robin had fallen from its nest. Well, I knew what to do. In Minnesota we take a cardboard box, fill it with grass and leaves, put the baby bird in it, and feed the baby bird a combination of oatmeal and skim milk through a medicine dropper. Armed with all the right stuff, I followed John to where the baby bird lay in the grass.

One look at the bird told me that it couldn't possibly make it. Its feathers were still wet. Clearly, it was far too premature to live. Gently, I told John that we would do the best we could. My exuberant son was leaping into the air exclaiming: "His name is Oscar." I cringed. It would be so much harder when the bird died now that it had a name.

We put Oscar in a safe place and went into the house for dinner. At bedtime, John said he wanted to remember Oscar in his prayers. I cringed again. I was his Sunday School teacher that year. We hadn't discussed how God answers prayers. We didn't discuss theology that night either. We prayed. Oscar made it.

Just before the strong, healthy little robin flew away from our neighborhood, he perched in a tree next to our garage. My neighbor came over and took a photo. That photograph is still on the freezer door of our refrigerator.

The photo of Oscar reminds us all of how little we know—that knowledge isn't really what is ultimately important. Faith is.

The diagnosis of diabetes, or any chronic disease, brings lots of questions. Why me? Why now? What does the future hold? Health care professionals can project—some even predict—but no one can "know" enough to answer these questions.

Living comfortably with unanswerable questions requires faith. Elie Wiesel, one of the best known Jewish writers, went through Auschwitz and wrote, "Heaven is the place where questions and answers become one."

A similar thought is expressed in the Christian tradition by the apostle Paul (1 Corinthians 13:12):

For now I see in a mirror dimly, but then face to face. Now I know in part; then I shall understand fully, even as I have been fully understood.

Where do you turn for comfort with your unanswerable questions?

The golden moments in the stream of life rush past us and we see nothing but sand; the angels come to visit us, and we only know them when they are gone.

–George Eliot

Do you believe in angels? On topics such as this, I listen to my heart to make my own decision, but my head also listens to people whom I respect. My friend Bob Esbjornson refers to angels as "messengers of El," the Hebraic idea of angel. The book of Hebrews has a statement about angels: "Do not neglect to show hospitality to strangers, for thereby some have entertained angels unawares." I have heard and read that statement many times over the years. I have wondered at its meaning. My own response has been, "But, I'm busy, and my house is a mess." I have only looked at the meaning literally, to mean people coming into my house.

Bob refers to messages as angels. The messengers can be the ideas in a book (read meditatively) or a movie or lecture (watched and listened to meditatively). He refers to authors as strangers to whom he opened his mind, hospitable to the message. He said, "It's a matter of being hospitable to strangers, to people with ideas that are unfamiliar to me but somehow connect with ideas at home in my mind."

Open my mind to welcome strangers.
Help me to see the angels.

A favorite print that my great-aunt had in her home showed two small children standing on a rickety, old bridge over a river. The little boy was leaning over precariously as if to retrieve a shiny stone. Unbeknownst to either child, an angel had her finger through the belt loop on the back of his trousers.

For he will give his angels charge of you to guard you in all your ways. On their hands they will bear you up, lest you dash your foot against a stone.

−Psalm 91:11-12

Although that is both a lovely and a comforting thought, I believe there is an important issue of self-responsibility, stewardship. I do believe in angels, but I also believe that I am expected to do the best I can to act responsibly and not demand that angels protect me when I am acting irresponsibly. This belief causes me to monitor my blood glucose levels often so that I can drive a car safely, exercise with plenty of "fuel," and keep my blood sugars in a range that will not harm my blood vessels.

Consider where you are on the angel issue as well as on your personal responsibility.

Emotional and spiritual healing is important if we are to be whole people. But, healing does not always just happen. Sometimes we need help to heal. Sometimes healing takes a long time.

Eight years after my son was born and seriously injured, I finally healed. The emotional pain ended. My pain was the result of my having "stuffed" my anger after he was injured. I told myself that it wasn't Christian to be angry. That thought helped to heap guilt on top of my pain.

There were two experiences that led to my healing. One was a sermon by one of our pastors who has a severely handicapped son. He told us that he literally shook his fist at God and asked, "Where were you?!" (Wow. I never dreamed that pastors got angry at God! That helped alleviate my feelings of guilt.) And, our pastor said that he felt the response of God was: "I was there . . . grieving with you."

The experience that clinched my healing occurred when I was invited to speak at a risk management conference to people very concerned about issues like malpractice lawsuits. I was invited because the physician in charge knew about my son's injury and the fact that we had never sued. He wanted me to share our story.

At the end of my presentation, I said, "There's one thing I don't understand. The hospital never apologized to my husband and me. Are hospitals so afraid of culpability that they cannot be human?" It was a rhetorical question. I stepped down from the podium. A man approached me and said, "I know the hospital that you're speaking of. I work there but wasn't there when your son was born. I'm eight years late, but on behalf of the hospital, I want to apologize to you and your husband." Tears of healing streamed down his face and mine.

My father-in-law immigrated to the United States from Norway as a young man. He met and married my mother-in-law, and they had the first of their three children. When World War II broke out, my father-in-law was drafted into the Army. When he returned to the U.S., he had a wife and daughter but no job. He wanted very much to be a carpenter but was told that he needed the union's permission to become an apprentice. The union refused permission because he was inexperienced and, at age 34, too old.

One day, my in-laws sat at their kitchen table discussing the situation. My father-in-law began to cry at the prospect of not being able to provide for his family. My mother-in-law looked at the unfamiliar and improbable sight of her husband weeping. She gathered her composure, focused on the source of their faith, and began to sing a familiar hymn. The soothing words of this hymn from childhood gave her strength.

Oh, what peace we often forfeit; Oh, what needless pain we bear.
All because we do not carry everything to God in prayer.

When she finished singing, she squared her shoulders and said: "You go back to the union and tell them all the experience that you *do* have. Then, you tell them that if you can fight for your country at age 34, you can certainly become a carpenter's apprentice." He went to the union, and the rest, as they say, is history. We attended the celebration when he was honored for 50 years in the carpenter's union.

Stories make tangible the intangible. *Faith* has many faces . . . my mother-in-law's is one of them.

Faith is a bird
Which feels the light
And sings in the dark
Before the dawn.

–Anonymous

Energy, for a variety of reasons, can become low in people who have diabetes. Low blood sugars can leave us feeling virtually lifeless. Beyond physical energy, it is spiritual energy that keeps us going on our darkest days through the roughest places on our walk.

What carbohydrate is to a low blood sugar, inspiring words are to the spirit.

They who wait for the Lord shall renew their
    strength,
they shall mount up with wings like eagles,
they shall run and not be weary,
they shall walk and not faint.

–Isaiah 40:31

Reading and rereading great literature is important because each reading can bring new meaning. The Psalms were my great-grandmother's favorite. I have her Bible, and the Psalms are tattered and torn from her rereading of this sacred and meaningful text. One of her four sons, my great-uncle Andrew was killed in World War I. The Psalms may be where she found comfort, strength, and peace.

When my son had surgery at the age of four, I was very concerned about the anesthesia. My concern centered around a mistaken dosage . . . too much anesthesia.

I found peace in Psalm 121:

The Lord will keep your going out and your coming in from this time forward and for evermore.

When people experience Life's toughest times, quite often they turn to the power they recognize as greater than they. The connection or reconnection is life transforming . . . the proverbial blessing in adversity.

Some people describe their experience as one of using the spiritual to help them transcend the reality of their pain. Others say that their painful experiences, as unwelcome as they are, help them to focus on what they truly value—spiritual values. So, the question seems to be: Are we transcending reality or ascending to reality?

We are not human beings having a spiritual experience. We are spiritual beings having a human experience.

–Pierre Teilhard de Chardin

Great stress is created when we feel pushed to respond to the commands and demands of others. At times we may even feel that our lives are controlled by tyrants. We can experience tyranny at work, at home, at medical appointments . . . Sorting through the various demands, we decide for ourselves what is important.

The only tyrant I accept in this world is the still small voice within me.
—Mahatma Gandhi

The kingdom of God is within you.
—Luke 17:21

The voice of God is always speaking to us and always trying to get our attention. But His voice is a "still, small voice," and we must at least slow down in order to listen.
—Eugenia Price

**Consider what you might gain
by losing your hectic pace of life.**

Within you, there exists a stillness and sanctuary to which you can retreat at any time and be yourself.
—Siddhartha

"The *Torah* wants me to stay healthy," says Rabbi Ave Boruch Hollander. In an article in the February 1997 *Diabetes Forecast* magazine, Hollander goes on to say, "That's why I take my diabetes regimen as seriously as I take my religion." An orthodox Jew, Hollander believes that *Torah*, the law of Moses, relates to every part of his life—including diabetes and diet. Illustrating this point, he explained: "*Torah* tells us that one good deed brings another, and that one sin brings another. And it's true.

"When I make one good food choice, odds are that I will make another good food choice. And, when I make a poor food choice, I usually follow it with another poor food choice." Hollander describes his interweaving of religion and health in this way: "*Torah* asks us to live in the real world. And food and health, and certainly diabetes, are in the real world."

Adding another dimension to Rabbi Hollander's view of religion, diabetes, and life is the Talmud (Jewish Oral Law). Hollander said, "The Talmud tells us that this world is a long narrow bridge and that we are all on it together, and it is up to us to help each other."

And what is his "real world" motivation? "I would like to be around to dance at my children's grandchildren's weddings."

Incline your ear, and come to me; hear, that your soul may live.

–Isaiah 55:3

Isaiah's ancient advice holds great insight into the nature of our spiritual life. The most obvious meaning in that passage is that as we read and listen to God's Word, we will be nourished spiritually. We will be spiritually alive.

I also understand in Isaiah's words that we are to listen to our hearts . . . where God resides. We are, in fact, to seek God everywhere and as we seek, we shall find.

With the intent of finding God, I can incline my ear to a flower . . . and find Him.

Help my soul to seek, to hear, and to live.

God calls us away from the tumult of the world,
that we may focus our lives on things that are
lasting. In God's presence we see our lives more
clearly; the broken pieces are put back together.
God calls us out of loneliness into a life of
community. Worshipping together, caring about
one another, we find out what it means to be
truly human.

—Pastor Terry Morehouse

A humble, informal church service in a rural setting began with this prayer that clearly explained why we were together on a "retreat." Community is a key component to healthy living. In community we know that we are not alone. We can receive support and give support.

Diabetes is one of many examples of the brokenness and isolation in the world. Support groups of the American Diabetes Association, local hospitals, clinics, and places of worship provide us the opportunity to create community and heal the brokenness. And, when we give to help one another to heal, we discover what it means to be truly human. We realize that we are not broken; we are whole.

In the PBS show *Amazing Grace with Bill Moyers*, Moyers interviewed country singer Johnny Cash about the song's power. Cash recalled having sung "Amazing Grace" to prison inmates. He said, "For the three minutes that song is sung, everyone's free."

Singer Judy Collins, who also recorded "Amazing Grace," told Moyers that when she sings it, there is a "mystical territory" between the song and audience. Finding a power all its own, the song heals.

I recall a difficult time in my life when I played Judy Collins' recording of "Amazing Grace" every day. For the several minutes that I listened to her singing, I experienced the freedom that Johnny Cash referred to and the healing Judy Collins recognized. I felt connected to the many thousands of people who, over the years, have listened to or sung this beautiful hymn and, taking spiritual refreshment from the song, have turned to meet adversity with courage and grace.

Bring me to the music that nourishes my spirit.

Spirit comes from a Greek word that can also mean breath or wind. We do not see wind any more than we see the spirit. But everywhere we can see the evidence that they exist.

Leaves swirl, branches sway—although we don't see the wind, we see what it does. What evidence exists for the spirit?

Page through the book of Life. Where have you seen, heard, or experienced any of these fruits of the spirit?

> *Love*
> *Joy*
> *Peace*
> *Patience*
> *Kindness*
> *Goodness*
> *Faithfulness*
> *Gentleness*
> *Self-Control*
>
> –Galatians 5:22

To show each of these fruits, give a story from your life that will make it real. Then you will see the evidence of the spiritual.

Each of us has a string of pearls . . . in our hearts. These "pearls" are the beautiful moments we've experienced thus far in life. These are moments that become memories that will:

> Uplift
> Enliven
> Gladden
> Soften
> Inspire
> Guide

There are plenty of baubles, bangles, and beads in life . . . only a few gems.

Close your eyes and "see" your string of pearls. Name the gems—by person, by place, by experience, by gift of the spirit.

Whether or not you wear jewelry . . . wear your spiritual string of pearls.

Our wholeness depends upon our ability to heal when we are broken. I listened deeply to a friend who had lost his wife of nearly 50 years.

He said she was not his center of value, his "god." Losing her, therefore, was not the same as losing ultimate value. He said that as important as marriage and family were to him, they were not his religion. Then came the statement that awakened my soul.

"I belong to a larger family, those who give the Lord glory and laud and honor." He said more after that but I was on a journey with the previous thought. I am part of a family that goes back to the very beginning and that will go forward until the proverbial end of the age.

Without remembering any previous lonely or sad feelings, I was suddenly and acutely aware of warm feelings, comfort, security . . . belonging to love, claimed by love, and understanding this love as unchanging and eternal.

"Thought" journeys can be pretty astounding.

Let everything that breathes praise the Lord!
–Psalm 150:6

In the Hebrew language, there is no word for "thank you." When thanks appear in Hebrew writing, the word used is the Hebrew word for praise.

What connection do you find between thanks and praise?

What is the "attitude of gratitude?"

Writer C.S. Lewis described praise as "inner health made audible."

What does inner health mean to you? What does it look like? Is it healthy organs? A healthy mind? A healthy spirit? What causes it to become "audible?"

Does its audible expression mean singing? Shouting? Laughing? Speaking in a whisper?

Consider . . . explore . . . enjoy your thoughts.

Sometimes our anguish is caused by a misunderstanding. Years ago I was in a Bible study. During our small group discussion one day, a woman blurted out: "I just can't be thankful for all circumstances!" She was referring to a scripture passage. But she misunderstood it.

Our group discussion leader calmly and gently spoke. (She had lost her five-year-old son to leukemia.) Beth said, "The actual passage reads: "Give thanks *in* all circumstances, not *for* all circumstances."

As Beth's words sank in, we watched the weight of the world lift from the woman's shoulders. It pays to ask questions. Sincere "seeking" is not disrespectful. The rewards can be great.

Cure vs. Heal

In today's health care, we are faced with growing (and already large) numbers of people who have chronic diseases. Diabetes is a chronic disease, that is, there is no cure for it. How we live with that fact directly affects the quality of our lives.

And, although a cure is not yet possible, healing is ever possible, and, in fact, healing can greatly enhance our quality of life.

Cure is a physical act. Healing is spiritual.

Consider where you are spiritually. Are you on a healing path? What signs in your life tell you that you are on a healing path? How do you measure and, therefore, evaluate your healing? Consider the following as you reflect on your life.

A healing path might include: engaging in meditation, having an active prayer life, discussing feelings, having a readily identifiable support network, journal-keeping, acknowledging the need to heal, and actively seeking healing.

Signposts along the healing path that indicate a measure of healing can include: feelings of peace, faith, hope, and courage; an attitude of acceptance rather than resignation; and the belief in your heart-of-hearts that your experience with diabetes has given you insights that you value.

What are they?

At my church, I facilitate a group comprised of people who have a chronic health challenge. Some have diabetes. Others have any of a large variety of challenges. It is not our individual health challenge that brings us together. It is our desire for "wholeness." We recognize that physical ailments cannot always be cured, but that healing is always a possibility . . . and we actively seek that healing.

I wrote the following prayer for this group. Consider it. Consider what additions or changes you would make so that it would speak for you.

Dear Lord,

>*We come before you seeking wholeness. Heal us as it is your will to do so. If total physical healing is not your Plan, then we pray for the grace and strength to accept our challenges.*
>
>*Grant us health and healing of our minds and spirits. May we have wisdom to live faithfully, love to give to all with whom we interact, joy in the many gifts You provide us daily, and peace forever in our hearts.*

Thank you, gracious Lord.
Amen.

Grief hollows us out that we may hold more joy.
                                              –Kahlil Gibran

The spiritual dimension of life is where we explore and find courage, joy, wisdom, faith, steadfastness, hope, and peace . . . among other spiritual qualities. Consider this thought and see where it leads you. Agree or disagree, but know what you think and why you think it.

Fear, stress, pain, and loss are our truest gifts because it is their presence that calls forth the spiritual qualities from deep within us.

What is *your* philosophy? What is your belief about suffering? How do you heal?

When I do my workout, I almost always include a brisk 30- to 40-minute walk for the aerobic part. As I walk, I pray. When I make the petition "Create in me a clean heart and renew within me a right spirit," I ask for clean arteries, veins, and capillaries. I ask that my heart be cleansed physically, emotionally, and spiritually.

As I ask for the renewal of a right spirit, I ponder recent events in my life. Identifying my shortcomings and weaknesses, I ask for strength.

Then, I listen.

Talking is the easy part. Listening is hard.
Sometimes the "still, small voice"
is very, very quiet.

Youth never despairs, for it is still in harmony
with the Divine.

—Alexandre Dumas

When our son was in second grade, he had a Sunday School teacher who assigned scripture to be memorized each week. One Sunday evening after checking the assignment sheet affixed to our refrigerator door, I told John that the week's memory verse was "Trust in God."

"Oh, good!" he said enthusiastically, "that's easy." My eyes immediately met my husband's as we nonverbally communicated our understanding that it is not "easy" to trust.

My next thought was that John meant that three words are easy to memorize. My lasting belief is that childlike faith does include an ease in trusting God. It is adulthood that creates "disease" or disharmony through disappointments that have not been reconciled.

For years I taught first grade Sunday School. I presented the weekly lesson. But I learned as much as I taught. The children provided the lasting lesson of trust.

We don't need to lose our childlike faith.

Music therapy is now a major course of study offered at some colleges. Schools are keying into what intuition has told us for centuries. Music has potent power to heal. In 1988, I gave the keynote address for the American Association of Diabetes Educators. I predicted that music would be part of our spiritual approach to healing. I jokingly predicted that diabetes educators might need signed, informed consent forms to play music as powerful as that of Neil Diamond.

The ultimate application of this musical therapy needs to be self-applied based on your unique needs and desires. Consider today the music that you like. Do you have several types that appeal to you for different reasons? Is there one that helps you manage stress, another that revitalizes your spirit, calms, energizes, or . . . . What are the ways you use music?

The best way with music, I imagine, is not to bring the forces of our intellect to bear upon it, but to be still and let it work on that part of us for whose sake it exists.

–George MacDonald

Diabetes is an unwelcome intruder in the lives of people who already have challenges with which they must cope. "Why me?" is a common question. "Why?" is also a common question found in the Psalms.

In his book, *Psalms for Sojourners*, James Limburg points us to some interesting thoughts about the Psalms. The question "Why?" is directed to God; the question is never answered. But the Psalms do not end with questions. They move to affirmations, and, in nearly all of them, the Psalms end with words of praise.

As we travel our journey with diabetes, we find many questions to explore. The fortunate among us find life-affirming experiences and fellow travelers that lift us when the questions have no answers. We are truly blessed if we can end our journey with words of praise.

Help me to be able to affirm life, my life.
May this experience with diabetes
be one of learning and growth.
May my final words be ones of praise.

The best and most beautiful things in the world cannot be seen or even touched. They must be felt with the heart.

–Helen Keller

The spiritual helps us to transcend what we can see, to believe what we cannot see. That's faith.

Evangelist Billy Graham commented once that although he does not understand the digestive system, he still eats. And, although he doesn't understand all about the respiratory system, still he continues to breathe. "And," he said, "So it is with faith."

Where do these thoughts take you? Can you recall experiences you've had when you rose above what was visible and felt a truth in your heart?

We shall not cease from exploration;
And the end of all exploring will be to arrive
where we started
And know the place for the first time.
–T.S. Elliott

Human development continues for all of our lifetime. We learn more about ourselves and the world each time we encounter one another. The process of gaining insight seems to require us to explore, reflect, apply, and evaluate.

Each review of familiar places and experiences on our exploration presents us with a new perspective. Thus it is that we can "arrive where we started and know the place for the first time." The place hasn't changed. We have.

This is a very hopeful thought. We can revisit pain and find lessons in peace. We can revisit jealousy and find cooperation and trust. We can revisit fear and find that what we ran away from before was courage disguised. And Joy cannot be sought and found. It can only be found . . . at the place where we started.

Though we travel the world over to find the
beautiful, we must carry it with us or we find it
not.
–Ralph Waldo Emerson

We do carry beauty with us. We all started out with it. Explore. Find.

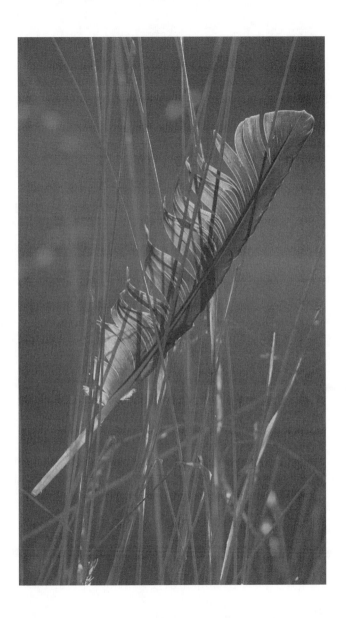

Epilogue

*Why does anybody tell a story? It does indeed
have something to do with faith, faith that the
universe has meaning, that our little human lives
are not irrelevant, that what we choose to say or
do matters, matters cosmically.*

–Madeleine L'Engle

I continue talking with God. Each day, many
times each day, I ask for guidance or I offer thanks.
And when I am truly wise, I listen.

As a seeker of meaning, I have come to understand that there are no answers to questions about
why tragedies befall us. Rather than answers to
"why," we receive responses when we ask "how."
We are given insights into how we can cope with
the challenges life presents, how we can weave
difficulty and joy into the tapestry of our lives.
Our worldview expands as we develop a philosophy that allows us to accept graciously both
tragedy and triumph. Life goes on—at first reluctantly, then the song returns to our hearts.

I have received an insight as a gift while writing this book: Although it has always been enormously helpful to be able to "hand over" my burdens to God, I gain the most when I give Him
my trust.

I believe it is fitting that the concluding thought in this book should come from my mentor and beloved friend, Bob Esbjornson. The thought is the last line in his book *Final Time*. I phrase it as a question to encourage your thinking and your seeking for meaning.

Is it possible that after we have traveled the valleys and the mountain tops through all the seasons of our lives, we shall experience "a glory beyond reason in a life beyond season?"

Blessings to you.

Self-Care

New!
When Diabetes Hits Home
Wendy Satin Rapaport, LCSW, PsyD
A reassuring exploration of the full spectrum
of emotional issues you and your family may struggle
with throughout your lives. You'll learn how to cope with
the initial period of anger and anxiety at diagnosis,
develop your spiritual self and discover the meaning of
living with a chronic disease, address the changes all
families go through and learn how to cope with them
emotionally, much more.
#4818-01   One Low Price: $19.95

New!
The Uncomplicated Guide to Diabetes Complications
Edited by Marvin E. Levin, MD and Michael A. Pfeifer, MD
Thorough, comprehensive chapters cover everything you
need to know about preventing and treating diabetes complications—in simple language that anyone can understand.
All major complications and special concerns are covered,
including kidney disease, heart disease, obesity, eye disease
and blindness, impotence and sexual disorders, hypertension
and stroke, neuropathy and vascular disease, more.
#4814-01   One Low Price: $18.95

New!
Caring for the Diabetic Soul
Simple solutions for coping with the psychological
challenges of diabetes.
#4815-01   Nonmember: $9.95   Member: $8.95

Bestseller!
ADA Complete Guide to Diabetes
Packed with ideas, tips, and techniques for dealing with
all types of diabetes.
#4809-01   Nonmember: $19.95   Member: $17.95

Revised Bestseller!

Type 2 Diabetes: Your Healthy Living Guide, 2nd Edition

A thorough guide to staying healthy with type 2 diabetes.
#4804-01   Nonmember: $16.95   Member: $14.95

New!

Women & Diabetes

Laurinda M. Poirier, RN, MPH, CDE and
Katherine M. Coburn, MPH
Special thoughts to help a diabetic woman move
through life with confidence.
#4907-01   Nonmember: $14.95   Member: $13.95

New!

The Commonsense Guide to Weight Loss

Barbara Caleen Hansen, PhD and
Shauna S. Roberts, PhD
Learn how to lose weight—and keep it off—using medically proven techniques from the weight-loss experts. You'll discover the seven crucial elements of weight loss for people with diabetes, including how to choose the right target weight; make permanent lifestyle changes; measure weight-loss progress by tracking health, not weight; develop a healthy meal plan; maintain an active lifestyle; more.   #4816-01   One Low Price: $19.95

New

The Complete Weight Loss Workbook

Judith Wylie-Rosett, EdD, RD, Charles Swencionis, PhD, Arlene Caban, BS, Allison J. Friedler, BS, and Nicole Schaffer, MA
Proven techniques for controlling weight-related health problems. The authors devised a unique workbook that offers a series of checklists, worksheets, mini-cases, calculation exercises, mental reminders, and other practical aids to knocking off those extra pounds and staying fit for good. Features real-life examples of people who illustrate and explain the patterns that lead to success or failure in watching your weight.   #4812-01   One Low Price: $17.95

Bestseller!

101 Tips for Improving Your Blood Sugar
David S. Schade, MD, and Associates
Dozens of tips for improving your blood sugar
and reducing your risk of complications.
#4805-01   Nonmember: $12.95   Member: $10.95

Cooking and Nutrition

Month of Meals: Classic Cooking
Choose from the classic tastes of Chicken Cacciatore,
Oven Fried Fish, Sloppy Joes, Shish Kabobs, Roast Leg
of Lamb, Lasagna, Minestrone Soup, Grilled Cheese
Sandwiches, many others. And just because it's Christmas doesn't mean you have to abandon your healthy
meal plan. A "Special Occasion" section offers tips for
brunches, holidays, parties, and restaurants to give you
delicious dining options in any setting. 58 pages.
Spiral-bound.   #4701-01   One Low Price: $14.95

Month of Meals: Ethnic Delights
A healthy diet doesn't have to keep you from enjoying
your favorite restaurants: tips for Mexican, Italian, and
Chinese restaurants are featured. Quick-to-fix and eth-
nic recipes are also included. Choose from Beef Burritos,
Chop Suey, Veal Piccata, Stuffed Peppers, and many
others. 63 pages. Spiral-bound.
#4702-01   One Low Price: $14.95

Month of Meals: Meals in Minutes
Eat at McDonald's, Wendy's, Taco Bell, and other fast
food restaurants and still maintain a healthy diet. Special sections offer tips on planning meals when you're
ill, reading ingredient labels, preparing for picnics and
barbeques, more. Quick-to-fix menu choices include
Seafood Stir Fry, Fajita in a Pita, Hurry-Up Beef Stew,
Quick Homemade Raisin Bread, Macaroni and Cheese,
many others. 80 pages. Spiral-bound.
#4703-01   One Low Price: $14.95

Month of Meals: Old-Time Favorites

Old-time family favorites like Meatloaf and Pot Roast will remind you of the irresistible meals grandma used to make. Hints for turning family-size meals into delicious "planned overs" will keep leftovers from going to waste. Meal plans for one or two people are also featured. Choose from Oven Crispy Chicken, Beef Stroganoff, Kielbasa and Sauerkraut, Sausage and Cornbread Pie, and many others. 74 pages. Spiral-bound.
#4704-01   One Low Price: $14.95

Month of Meals: Vegetarian Pleasures

Choose from a garden of fresh selections like Eggplant Italian, Stuffed Zucchini, Cucumbers with Dill Dressing, Vegetable Lasagna, and many others. Craving a snack? Try Red Pepper Dip, Eggplant Caviar, or Beanito Spread. A special section shows you the most nutritious ways to cook with whole grains, and how to add flavor to your meals with peanuts, walnuts, pecans, pumpkin seeds, and more. 58 pages. Spiral-bound.
#4705-01   One Low Price: $14.95

New!
The Diabetes Snack Munch Nibble Nosh Book
Ruth Glick

Choose from 150 low-sodium, low-fat snacks and mini-meals such as pizza puffs, mustard pretzels, apple-cranberry turnovers, bread puzzle, cinnamon biscuits, pecan buns, alphabet letters, banana pops, and many others. Special features include recipes for one or two and snack ideas for hard-to-please kids. Nutrient analyses, preparation times, and exchanges are included with every recipe.
#4622-01   One Low Price: $14.95

About the American Diabetes Association

The American Diabetes Association is the nation's leading voluntary health organization supporting diabetes research, information, and advocacy. Founded in 1940, the Association provides services to communities across the country. Its mission is to prevent and cure diabetes and to improve the lives of all people affected by diabetes.

For more than 50 years, the American Diabetes Association has been the leading publisher of comprehensive diabetes information for people with diabetes and the health care professionals who treat them. Its huge library of practical and authoritative books for people with diabetes covers every aspect of self care—cooking and nutrition, fitness, weight control, medications, complications, emotional issues, and general self care. The Association also publishes books and medical treatment guides for physicians and other health care professionals.

Membership in the Association is available to health care professionals and people with diabetes and includes subscriptions to one or more of the Association's periodicals. People with diabetes receive *Diabetes Forecast*, the nation's leading health and wellness magazine for people with diabetes. Health care professionals receive one or more of the Association's five scientific and medical journals.

For more information, please call toll-free:

Questions about diabetes:	1-800-DIABETES
Membership, people with diabetes:	1-800-806-7801
Membership, health professionals:	1-800-232-3472
Free catalog of ADA books:	1-800-232-6733
Visit us on the Web:	www.diabetes.org
Visit us at our Web bookstore:	merchant.diabetes.org